Fabiana Gonçalves Seki Gava

Bach Flower Therapy for Stress Reduction

Fabiana Gonçalves Seki Gava

Bach Flower Therapy for Stress Reduction

Clinical Trial Conducted with Primary Health Care Nursing Professionals

ScienciaScripts

Imprint

Any brand names and product names mentioned in this book are subject to trademark, brand or patent protection and are trademarks or registered trademarks of their respective holders. The use of brand names, product names, common names, trade names, product descriptions etc. even without a particular marking in this work is in no way to be construed to mean that such names may be regarded as unrestricted in respect of trademark and brand protection legislation and could thus be used by anyone.

Cover image: www.ingimage.com

This book is a translation from the original published under ISBN 978-620-6-76150-1.

Publisher:
Sciencia Scripts
is a trademark of
Dodo Books Indian Ocean Ltd. and OmniScriptum S.R.L publishing group

120 High Road, East Finchley, London, N2 9ED, United Kingdom
Str. Armeneasca 28/1, office 1, Chisinau MD-2012, Republic of Moldova, Europe
Printed at: see last page
ISBN: 978-620-7-93554-3

INTRODUCTION

The COVID-19 pandemic has generated a political, economic, social and health system crisis in the country, with an increased sense of insecurity, uncertainty and lack of control, triggering psychological distress in individuals[1]. The social isolation caused by quarantine, loneliness, physical distance from friends and family, fear and grief can lead to the development of psychological problems and the worsening of mental and emotional disorders[2]. Psychological disorders have been observed during the pandemic at individual, community, national and global levels[3].

In addition to the factors common to the general population, there are also those that are specific to health professionals who worked during the pandemic, such as the risk of contamination, the lack of protective equipment, work overload, discrimination, frustration and exhaustion[4]. During this period, a high prevalence of depression, anxiety and stress was observed in all health professional categories[1]. In nursing, which is the category that spends the most time directly caring for patients[5], the prevalence of stress according to a meta-analysis carried out in 2021 was 43%[6]. In Brazil, a study carried out in the same year found a 49% prevalence of stress among these professionals[1].

The physical and mental health disorders caused by stress lead to

the burden on the health system and society worldwide. Individuals who suffer from stress-related illnesses see doctors three to five times more often and are hospitalised six times more often than people who don't suffer from these conditions[7].

Stress has deleterious effects on the nervous, immune, cardiovascular, digestive, endocrine systems and the brain-intestine axis, leading to the development of pathologies associated with these systems, such as reduced memory, cognition and learning; behavioural and mood disorders; growth of malignant cells, instability genetic and tumour growth, a chronic increase in inflammatory processes or a state of immunosuppression; atherosclerosis, arrhythmias and acute myocardial infarction; Crohn's disease, ulcerative diseases and irritable bowel syndrome, among others[8-9].

As a result of stress, individuals can adopt unhealthy health behaviours such as low levels of physical activity, smoking and alcohol and drug abuse, which can compromise family and social relationships[5]. There are also labour repercussions such as low motivation, reduced job satisfaction, intention to leave work or change profession, low productivity, high turnover, absenteeism and presenteeism[10].

Because of all its harmful effects, it is necessary to develop efficient strategies for individuals to manage situations they consider stressful. Integrative and complementary health practices (ICPHPs) such as meditation, acupuncture, yoga, aromatherapy and flower therapies have been used to help cope with these situations, either on their own or in support of other therapies[5].

Because it takes a holistic approach to the human being in its physical, emotional, mental, social and spiritual dimensions[11], flower therapy focuses on helping the individual to regain their balance, in an individualised way, so that they can carry out the healing process themselves. The use of this therapy has been recognised and recommended by the World Health Organisation since 1956, and has been regulated for use in Brazil's Unified Health System by the National Policy for Integrative and Complementary Health Practices - PNPIC[12-13]. Bach florals are a simple, low-cost alternative with no side effects that can be used concomitantly with other interventions as an auxiliary strategy for stress management. Based on the above, the question that this he research aims to answer is: are Bach florals effective in reducing stress in primary health care nursing professionals?

Based on the premise that flower therapy can help reduce stress, the hypothesis of this study is H1: Flower therapy is effective in reducing stress in primary health care nursing professionals.

Stress

Work can be a source of suffering or pleasure[14]. It is a fundamental element in the construction of the human being, not only because of its survival aspect, but also because of its possibilities for personal and professional fulfilment, as well as the possibility of technical, political, cultural, aesthetic and artistic training for the worker[14-15]. Work is a generator of health or illness, it is never neutral[14].

The great difficulty in differentiating occupational stress from general stress is that it is not possible to separate the inside of work from the outside of work, given that psychological functioning is not divisible. Mental setbacks are carried over from the work environment to the family environment and vice versa[14]. It is difficult to establish whether the consequences of stress are due to organisational stressors, events in the individual's life or a combination of both[16-17]. Good family and personal relationships have an impact on work and good work relationships have an impact on family and personal life[14].

Healthcare careers are considered inherently stressful due to long working hours, often poor working conditions, as well as difficulties in dealing with the severity of patients, pain and the finiteness of the human condition[18]. Higher levels of occupational stress have been observed in nursing staff for decades, as they are the professionals who spend the most time in direct patient care[5].

Due to the demanding and specific characteristics of the work process It is almost impossible to avoid stressors. For this reason, it is necessary to develop coping strategies with these teams so that stress does not affect performance and professional satisfaction[18], the physical and psychological health of professionals[19] and patient safety. Stress causes a decline in cognitive performance, in the ability to stay focused and process information, resulting in reduced alertness and decreased professional performance, which can threaten patients' lives and increase the risk of adverse medical events[20].

Stress is present at all levels of health care. Primary health care (PHC) presents stressors that are particular to this model of care, since its work processes differ from those of the hospital sector. The elements that contribute to the increased workload in PHC are: the complexity and excess of demands, the overestimated territory, the multiple activities provided for in the model, the excessive working hours, management failures, role ambiguity (taking on work that belongs to no one), lack of commitment from team members, staff shortages, shortages and precariousness of materials, structure and environment, and problems in resolving problems[21].

In addition to these elements, the way health is carried out in PHC exposes workers to very specific occupational risks. Home visits expose workers to the elements of nature, extremes of temperature, exposure to cigarette and vehicle smoke, and the risk of accidents such as falls, bites from venomous animals, dog bites, electric shock from contact with inadequate wiring and visits to homes at risk of collapse. The psychosocial risks most often mentioned by professionals include psychological overload due to not being able to comply with the working principles of PHC (universality, accessibility, linkage, continuity, accountability and humanisation), as well as pressure from users themselves, who don't understand this proposal for care, preferring models promotion and prevention models. Another important stressor is violence, since most basic units are located in peripheral areas with high rates of violence due to the presence of drug trafficking[22].

The concept of stress was initially studied by physics and engineering as an attribute of a material that undergoes the action of forces, and how much it can withstand these forces before breaking. During the Industrial Revolution in the 18th and 19th centuries, this concept came to have a connotation of force, effort and tension[23]. It was only in the 19th century that the concept of stress began to form part of the biological sciences. At that time, Claude Barnard described the processes of the internal environment of living beings, which must be kept stable and within parameters suitable for cellular function independent of the external environment, this being the ultimate function of all physiological mechanisms[8]. In the 20th century, Walter Cannon called the process discovered by Barnard homeostasis, and it was this concept that underpinned the biological model of stress described by Hans Selye in 1925[23].

Selye called the General Adaptation Syndrome (GAS) the body's physiological defence reaction in response to physical stimuli such as cold, heat, trauma, bleeding and infection. The GAS is made up of three phases. The Alarm Phase occurs immediately after the confrontation with the aggressor and has the function of defending the organism against situations that threaten its physical integrity. The Resistance Phase occurs if the stressor persists, and its aim is for the body to survive and adapt to the stressor. When the stressor persists and the body does not adapt to it, the Exhaustion Phase occurs, which is similar to the Alarm Phase, but more intense, and in the long term can lead to physical and mental illness and, in extreme cases, death[23]. SAG reactions occur due to the neuroendocrine response to the stressor, which involves two main axes: the sympathetic autonomic nervous system (SNAS) and the hypothalamic-pituitary axis (HPA). pituitary-adrenal (HPA). These two systems modulate a third, the immune system[24].

The SNAS is activated immediately when stressful events occur. This activation causes peripheral vasoconstriction, an increase in blood pressure, dilation of the bronchi and pupils and induction of the activity of the adrenal glands, which release the catecholamines adrenaline and noradrenaline. These hormones will stimulate skeletal muscle metabolism and central nervous system responses, leading to a general state of behavioural and cognitive alertness, preparing the individual for fight or flight[24].

When the HPA axis is activated, corticotrophin-releasing factor is initially released, which induces the synthesis and release of adrenocorticotrophic hormone in the adenohypophysis, which in turn induces the synthesis and release of glucocorticoids, cortisol being the main representative of this class of substances in primates. Cortisol induces systemic responses such as an increase in glycaemia, directing energy to sensory, cognitive and motor functions (essential in situations of challenge/threat), as well as stimulating the functioning of the cardiovascular and respiratory systems and inhibiting digestion, growth, reproduction and the perception of pain[24].

The immune system modulates the stress response through the release of cytokines, which can exert stimulatory or inhibitory effects on the SNAS and the HPA axis. The release of catecholamines stimulates the production of neutrophils and natural killer cells of the innate immune system, and the proliferation of cytotoxic T lymphocytes of the acquired immune system, which allows protection against infections arising from the stress response. Cortisol at moderate levels induces redistribution and displacement of lymphocyte production, helping to return the immune system to baseline levels[24].

Although the biological model has made significant contributions for the study of stress, it was criticised for its emphasis on the neuroendocrine impact, which does not take into account the response of individuals to stressful events and the psychological nature of stress. With the need to understand the emotional disorders of war veterans, the interactionist model of stress emerged in the 1960s. These investigations revealed that people respond differently to stressors and that, in addition to the physiological response, there is also a cognitive response to stress[23]. This approach takes into account personal and contextual variables involved in the situation and allows the encounter between the individual and the environment to be analysed, since in some situations considered stressful there are human variations, so that not all people experience stress, or experience it in the same way and with the same intensity[25].

In the interactionist model, the intensity of the biological response is influenced by the cognitive evaluation process, which activates the individual's cognitive, emotional and behavioural functions in relation to the stressor[23]. Stress is assessed by considering the stimulus (potentially stressful situation), the processes or responses (emotional or behavioural reactions to the stressor), and the results[25]. A representative of this model is Lazarus and the Cognitive Theory of Psychological Stress and Coping. According to this theory, stress is conceptualised as the relationship between the individual and the environment, which is evaluated by the person as threatening or challenging, and which exceeds their resources and puts their well-being at risk[26-27].

The Cognitive Theory of Psychological Stress and Coping was the theoretical framework adopted in this study. According to this theory, stress is mediated by cognitive evaluation and coping processes[25,28].

Coping relates to the cognitive and behavioural strategies used to manage internal and external demands that are assessed as stressful[27]. Coping has two main functions: managing the problem t h a t is causing the stress (problem-focused coping) and regulating the negative emotions and distress caused by the stressor (emotion-focused coping). Research shows that people use both strategies to deal with stressful situations[27,29]. A third type of coping was later added, meaning-focused coping, which regulates positive emotions[30].

Cognitive appraisal is the process by which the individual evaluates whether the stressful event is relevant to their well-being and, if so, in what way. There are three types of cognitive appraisal. In primary appraisal, the person attributes meaning to the event. Primary appraisal is influenced by factors such as the individual's values, beliefs and goals. If the person identifies the event as potentially harmful and threatening, they begin the secondary appraisal, in which they choose coping strategies for the situation in order to minimise the harm and increase the benefits[27,29]. The third type of assessment, called a reassessment, is carried out after the primary and secondary assessments, with the aim of understanding the situations and defining new forms of action, thus restarting the process[25].

Primary and secondary evaluations are influenced by social and personal resources. These factors influence both the definition of the type of event and the coping strategy to be used. Social resources include social support and material resources that give access to goods and services such as legal assistance, medical care and access to other professionals. Personal resources include those of a physical nature (health, energy levels), competences (social and problem-solving skills) and psychological resources (positive beliefs and values such as hope and spirituality)[25-26].

Spirituality derives from the word spiritus, or spirit in Latin. The spirit is the essential part of an individual, it controls the mind, and the mind controls the body. The spirit is the vital force that brings motivation and influences the life, health, behaviour and relationships[31].

Spirituality can be defined as an individual's propensity or set of beliefs that seeks meaning in life through a relationship with the transcendent[32], a sense of connection with something greater than oneself[33], which transmits vitality and meaning to life events[34], and which may or may not be linked to the sacred and religion[35].

There is scientific evidence associating religion and spirituality with different positive physical and mental health outcomes. On a physical level, they are related to lower hospitalisation rates, lower levels of pain, higher survival rates, better functionality in activities of daily living and better cardiovascular outcomes. In terms of mental health, they are associated with less development of depressive symptoms, lower rates of suicide and substance use, as well as protecting against the development of post-traumatic stress[36]. Religion and other spiritual interventions are reported to be effective means of coping with physical and mental stress[37].

There is a positive association between levels of spirituality and adaptation to stress[34]. In times of crisis, spirituality serves as a vital force that transmits hope e motivation[31]. Spiritual activitiespromote relief from fears and worries, bringing meaning, purpose and focus to the small joys of everyday life[38].

The essence of spirituality is the so-called numinous experience, which is unique to each individual. The numinous experience is a complex state of personal incompleteness associated with the desire to make contact with a higher power and find existential meaning. A crisis situation can make the individual aware of their incompleteness, leading them to search for meaning in their life. As a consequence, spirituality, as a form of coping, can help to transcend and reach a higher power, resulting in empowerment and increased abilities to deal with stressful situations[31]. Spirituality serves as a shield that protects against the adverse effects of everyday stressors. There is a a significant negative correlation between spiritual well-being and perceived stress[38].

Bach Flower Therapy

Bach flower therapy was systematised by the English physician Dr Edward Bach in 1928[12]. The flower essences used in this therapy are composed of substrates which, under the action of heat, are transmitted to the water in which the flowers are immersed[12,39].

Flowers act on the balance of individuals, bringing harmony, stabilising emotions and promoting a general sense of well-being[12,40-41]. There are no reports of side effects or addiction related to flower therapy, so there are no contraindications to its use. They can be used at all stages of human development and act on a preventative and curative level[42-43].

Bach flower therapy has 38 essences with specific indications, 37 of which are remedies based on wild flowers and trees, and one remedy prepared from the water of a natural spring with healing properties, as well as the emergency formula, also known as Rescue Remedy®, Five Flower® and Revival®[44].

The 38 Bach florals have been grouped into seven groups that represent the fundamental human conflicts that cause disharmony[45-47]:

• For those who feel afraid - essences that bring courage: Aspen, Cherry Plum, Mimulus, Red Chestnut, Rock Rose.

• For those suffering from insecurity or indecision - essences that promote decisiveness, assertiveness, confidence, surrender, hope and faith: Cerato, Gentian, Gorse, Hornbeam, Scleranthus, Wild Oat.

• For lack of interest in current circumstances - essences that bring focus and presence to the present moment: Chestnut Bud, Clematis, Honeysuckle, Mustard, Olive, White Chestnut, Wild Rose.

• For loneliness - essences that favour balance in relationships with personal rhythms: Heather, Impatiens, Water Violet.

• For those who are hypersensitive to influences and opinions - essences that help protect against limiting beliefs and aid in periods of transition: Agrimony, Centaury, Holly, Walnut.

• For despair - essences that bring encouragement in difficult and challenging situations: Crab Apple, Elm, Larch, Oak, Pine, Star of Bethlehem, Sweet Chestnut, Willow.

• For concern and excessive care for the well-being of others - essences that help you care for others and yourself with compassion: Beech, Chicory, Rock Water, Vervain, Vine.

As Dr Bach believed that all illness originated in the mind, which is the most delicate and sensitive part of the body, the 38 remedies correspond to the 38 mental states that predispose the individual to develop illnesses, whether physical or mental. In his writings on the 12 healers, Dr Bach says:

When caring for patients with these remedies, the nature of the illness is not taken into account; the individual is treated and, when they get better, their illness is gone, because it is expelled by the return of health (Bach, 2006, p. 71)

We all know that the same illness can have different effects on different people; it's the effects that we should be concerned with, because they lead us to true cause of the illness (Bach, 2006, p. 71).

This is why flower essences are not indicated for treating pathologies. There is no flower essence that can treat depression, for example. However, you can treat the emotional state that led to the disharmony and generated the depressive symptoms in that individual.

There is still no explanation of the mechanism of action of Bach florals[48]. Among the many theories about how they work, the most robust concerns nanoparticles (NP). Dr Edward Bach was a homeopathic doctor who integrated the basic and modified principles of homeopathy to develop flower therapy. Like homeopathy, flower essences also go through the process of ultra dilution for their manufacture, but they do not go through the process of succussion, which consists of intense agitation of the preparation in a glass vial. The preparations resulting from both therapies are also preserved in a mixture of water and ethanol called a mother tincture[49].

There have already been studies proving the presence of NPs in homeopathic medicines[50-51]. Although there are still no studies proving the presence of NPs in flower essences, due to their similarities with homeopathy, it can be inferred that Bach flower essences also contain NPs, which would explain their mechanism of action[52].

Nanoparticles are physical substrates that can carry information[53]. They are very small particles of material of natural or manufactured origin, and their size can vary from one to 1,000 nanometres[54]. NPs differ from the original bulk substances in their electromagnetic, optical, thermal, quantum and adsorption properties[54-55]. It is expected that the smallest NPs will be able to move around the body via the bloodstream or lymphatic system and cross cell membranes, including the blood-brain barrier, being able to carry out their functions inside cells[55].

NPs are biologically more potent forms than bulk substances. This is possible due to hormesis, a dose-response phenomenon in which a small stimulus leads to an increased response. Hormesis occurs through individual variations in the size, shape and charge of the particle surface. Another important point is that nano-drugs remain inside cells for longer than traditional medications. It is also known that the same dose of NPs, administered to different organisms, causes different effects, which justifies the need for adjustments due to individual characteristics in both homeopathy and flower therapy[54-55].

Several studies have proven the efficacy of Bach flower essences in maintaining the mental, psychological, emotional and even physical health of people of all ages.In a retrospective study of 41 clinical cases aimed at verifying the potential of Bach florals with an individualised formula for pain relief, 88% of participants showed an improvement in emotional well-being and 46% showed pain relief, which could be associated with improved stress levels, since there is a significant association between stress and increased pain[56].

The external use of Bach florals in a cream formulation was evaluated in a pilot study with carpal tunnel syndrome patients scheduled for surgery. The patients were randomly allocated to three groups: two blinded (placebo and Bach flower) and one group that received the flower formula unblinded. The flower formula was made up of five essences: Elm, Clematis, Star of Bethlehem, Vervain and Hornbeam and was used for 21 days. The results showed a beneficial effect of the flower on referred pain, nocturnal pain, tingling and numbness and an improvement in the signs of Phalen and Durcan with a large effect size, except for numbness. The authors emphasised as important aspects of the study the diagnostic assessment carried out by doctors, and the decrease in the number of patients who used flowers and required surgery compared to placebo[57].

Bach florals can help with altered childhood behaviour, such as tantrums, fits of rage, biting, screaming, banging one's head and holding one's breath[58]. In an experience report, the benefit of using a flower formula made up of four essences (Rescue Remedy®, Cherry Plum, White Chestnut and Walnut) was observed in the reduction and control of behaviours typical of the autistic spectrum in a seven-year-old child after 14 days of using the formula[59].

A cross-sectional study carried out with children aged six to seven showed that 82 per cent of them improved their fear of dentists after 30 days of using a Bach flower formula. The emergency flower was prescribed for seven days before starting treatment, followed by a formula with the essences Agrimony and Star of Bethlehem plus a flower specific to the child's fear: Aspen (unknown fear) or Mimulus (known fear)[60].

A randomised clinical trial carried out with nursing students indicated that those with high levels of state anxiety on the State-Trait Anxiety Inventory (SSTI) benefited from the use of Bach's emergency formula in reducing situational anxiety prior to taking academic exams[61]. Another randomised clinical trial carried out with workers showed that the formula made up of the essences Impatiens, White Chestnut, Cherry Plum and Beech promoted a statistically significant reduction in anxiety levels, when compared to placebo, after two months of treatment[62].

A descriptive, prospective study of men aged between 41 and 65 with andropause-related symptoms reported an improvement in the frequency of psychological symptoms such as anxiety (92.5%), apathy (92.3%), depression and irritability (83.3% both) with the use of individualised flower formulas[63].

A case report with two patients being treated for major depressive disorder showed a reduction in Beck Depression Inventory scores with the use of individualised flower formulas associated with psychotherapy and antidepressant medication, after 12 weeks of treatment[64].

A descriptive cross-sectional study was carried out with women who suffered psychological abuse determined the effectiveness of the individualised flower formula associated with psychological counselling in reducing negative emotional symptoms after three months of treatment[65]. A case report of the use of Bach florals in a patient with a history of sexual abuse, who was unable to establish a romantic relationship, evolved in such a way that, after four months of treatment with an individualised and adjusted formula, the patient reported significant improvements in her emotional well-being and, because she felt safe, she was able to start a romantic relationship[40].

Therapeutic intervention with florals carried out on chronic male alcoholics showed a satisfactory improvement (more than 80% reduction) in 93.3% of the patients in their psychosomatic manifestations, such as hypobulia, tremors, anxiety, anorexia, insomnia, decreased libido and alcohol intake. The formula used varied according to the psychosomatic condition presented, and could contain the essences Agrimony, Cherry Plum, Chicory, Impatiens, Walnut, Mimulus, Clematis, Scleranthus, Star of Bethlehem and the emergency formula[66].

A descriptive and exploratory qualitative study of parturient women concluded that the use of the emergency formula during the active phase of normal labour provided calm, relaxation, concentration and courage, which enabled these women to better control their pain[67]. Randomised clinical trial to measure the effectiveness of therapy flower essence in the reduction of repetitive and unwanted thoughts showed significant differences in favour of the floral group compared to placebo, with a medium effect size[68].

A study carried out in Taiwan that aimed to assess the effects of the emergency formula on the autonomic response of women subjected to a challenging mental situation found that those who received the flower had a significantly lower average heart rate variability when compared to participants who received a placebo[69].

A study of Brazilian primary school teachers, which used individualised formulas for each participant, showed significant results in reducing the stress of these professionals as measured by the List of Signs and Symptoms[70].

Randomised clinical trial carried out with overweight patients and obese people using the formula Impatiens, White Chestnut, Cherry Plum, Chicory, Crab Apple and Pine showed a significant reduction in the group that received the intervention in the outcomes anxiety, sleep quality, binge eating and resting heart rate, compared to the placebo group, after four weeks of use [52].

Good results in flower research have also been found in experimental research on animal models. A study on the central effects of Bach flower essences on mice showed antidepressant effects with Gorse essence, hypnotic effects with the formula composed of White Chestnut, Agrimony and Vervain essences, and anxiolytic effects with Agrimony essence[39].

Another study aimed to evaluate the effects of using preventive formula in the control of cardiovascular risk factors, showed that the rats that received florals had effective control of glycaemia, triglycerides and HDL cholesterol compared to the rats that did not receive the therapy[41].

A third pre-clinical, randomised, double-blind, placebo-controlled study aimed to evaluate the effect of flower essences on the in acute inflammation in rats with drug-induced plantar oedema, concluded that the flower essences showed anti-inflammatory activity with significant differences from placebo, with the Beech essence showing an immediate effect and the Vervain essence showing a delayed effect on inflammation[71].

More recently, in a randomised controlled clinical trial carried out on rats, the animals in the flower group that received the emergency formula showed a statistically significant reduction in their urea, glycaemia and alkaline phosphatase levels[72].

Although clinical practice shows very good results with the use of studies don't always reflect these results, which leads many researchers to conclude that flower therapy only works as a placebo. A randomised clinical trial carried out with psychiatric patients showed no difference between the placebo group and the intervention group in the use of floral therapy. emergency formula for controlling anxiety[73].

Another randomised clinical trial carried out with university students using the emergency formula found no significant difference between the intervention group and placebo for the test anxiety outcome[74].

Another randomised clinical trial that found no significant differences between the placebo group and the intervention group in reducing test anxiety in students used a formula made up of 10 essences: Impatiens, Mimulus, Gentian, Chestnut Bud, Rock Rose, Larch, Cherry Plum, White Chestnut, Scleranthus and Elm.[75]

A randomised clinical trial with nursing students aimed at evaluating the efficacy of the flower formula made up of the essences Cerato, Cherry Plum, Elm, Impatiens, Larch, Olive and White Chestnut in reducing stress found no significant results between the study groups as assessed by the Baccaro test[76].

A systematic review of five randomised clinical trials related to the use of flower therapy (with no defined outcome) published in 2010, concluded that there is no difference between flower therapy and placebo[77].

Another systematic review of randomised clinical trials published in 2009 analysed whether flower therapy was safe and effective in the treatment of psychological disorders and pain, and found no benefit for these conditions with the use of flowers compared to placebo groups[78].

OBJECTIVE

General objective

To evaluate the effectiveness of Bach flower therapy in relation to placebo in reducing levels of perceived stress in PHC nursing professionals.

Specific objectives

1. To describe the biosociodemographic profile of the participants.

2. To evaluate the effectiveness of the flower formula in reducing levels of perceived stress.
3. To evaluate the effectiveness of the floral formula in improving mood.

4. To assess the participants' perception of the use of the flower formula on their psycho-emotional states.
5. To assess the influence of coping strategies on reducing levels of perceived stress and improving mood.
6. To assess the influence of spirituality on reducing levels of perceived stress and improving mood.

METHOD

This is a pragmatic, parallel two-arm, double-blind, placebo-controlled randomised clinical trial (RCT) carried out from August 2021 to June 2022. The RCT is a quantitative, prospective and comparative study carried out under controlled conditions, in which interventions are randomly allocated to compare groups. When planned and conducted appropriately, the clinical trial is considered the most robust research method for determining the cause and effect relationship between an intervention and an outcome[79]. In this study, in order to bring the clinical trial closer to the daily lives of individuals, we opted for the pragmatic RCT, which allows for a population sample with less restrictive characteristics. The study scored 34 points in the PRagmatic Explanatory Continuum Indicator Summary (PRECIS-2) tool, which classifies it as a pragmatic clinical trial[80]. Pragmatic clinical trials are used to determine the effectiveness of an intervention in a scenario closer to real life. Unlike explanatory trials, pragmatic trials seek to ensure that the population studied is as similar as possible to the population in which the intervention will be applied. In addition, the interventions are more flexible and subject to modification, and the outcomes studied usually have clinical relevance for the research participants[81]. The project's registration in the PRECIS-2 tool is available for consultation at https://www.precis-2.org/Trials. The study followed the CONSORT (Consolidated Standards of Reporting Trials) recommendations for reporting clinical trials.

Location

The study was carried out in 32 of the 40 Basic Health Units (UBS) of the municipality of Osasco (São Paulo, Brazil), and at the School Health Centre Geraldo de Paula Souza (CSEGPS), in the municipality of São Paulo (São Paulo, Brazil). The CSEGPS was included in an attempt to reach the sample stipulated for the study.

Population

The population was made up of nurses, nursing assistants and technicians who worked in the UBS.
The inclusion criteria were self-reported stress, working at the institution for at

least six months, agreeing to take part in the study and using the treatment bottle as indicated.

The exclusion criteria were self-reported alcoholism (due to the presence of alcohol in the formulas) and being on holiday or away from work during the data collection period; using other ICPs during the research (individuals who use integrative practices may have positive expectations about the use of other ICPs, which may interfere with the study results[82].

Sampling

The sample calculation used information from the study by Pinto et al (2020)[70] which evaluated the effect of Bach flower therapy on reducing stress in teachers using the Perceived Stress Scale. Considering the effect size of the longitudinal difference f = 1.88, and for an effect of this magnitude to be declared significant with type I and II errors of 5%, test power = 80% and 95% confidence interval in an ANOVA model for repeated measures, it would be necessary to observe at least nine participants in total with all measurements, and the number of 50 participants in each study group was determined in case there was a need for stratified analyses.

Randomisation, allocation and masking

The vials were randomised simply, without blocking.

Each participant was identified by a number and the randomisation list was created in the Research Randomizer programme. The randomisation list was delivered in a sealed envelope and saved as a file on Google Drive. The researcher only had access to the physical and virtual list once the data collection had been finalised. To ensure blinding in both randomisation and the packaging of the vials, the identification process was carried out by an independent researcher who had no active role in applying the data collection instruments or distributing the vials. Neither the participants nor the researcher were aware of whether the bottle they received contained the placebo formula or the flower formula, as both were identical in flavour and appearance.

Loss of participants

Losses included participants who left the study on their own initiative after receiving the bottle, and participants who were excluded because they were away from work, either on sick leave, holiday or premium leave.

Even though participants were lost, the statistical analysis used allowed for the inclusion of individuals who did not complete the study. Therefore, the data of all participants who met the eligibility criteria and received the bottle were included in the data analysis.

Study and intervention groups

In 2019, a qualitative study was carried out with nursing professionals from a teaching hospital to identify how they perceived occupational stress through focus groups. The statements were grouped into five thematic categories: overload, physical tiredness, worry, self-blame, etc. and interpersonal relationships, which made it possible to propose the formula composed of the flower essences Elm, Olive, White Chestnut, Rock Water and Walnut.

Given the circumstances arising from the COVID-19 pandemic, the possibility of carrying out the research in hospital environments was restricted and the study site had to be changed. Based on the empirical experience of the researcher in the PHC environment, and drawing a parallel with the perception of professionals in the hospital environment of the research carried out, the flowers in the formula previously obtained were adjusted so that they portrayed the emotional state in the care environment of the COVID-19 pandemic[2,83]. In this context, the essence Rock Water was removed from the formula, and the flowers Cherry Plum and Star of Bethlehem were added.

Cherry Plum was indicated for the extreme situation that professionals were subjected to because of the pandemic, to restore lucidity in difficult times[67], pacify feelings and bring back the harmony that was broken by this event[44].

Elm is related to the principle of responsibility. The pandemic has brought extreme demands that have left professionals overburdened, both by responsibility and labour pressures, and by the increase in workload and volume[48,78]. Elm is also indicated for fatigue-related stress[12].

Hornbeam is indicated for tiredness that is more mental than physical, for those who lack the strength to fulfil their daily tasks[56]. People who need this essence lack the energy to fulfil their obligations, carrying out their work unwillingly, without pleasure and often procrastinating[48,78].

Olive's principle is that of regeneration[63]. This essence is indicated for periods of exhaustion as a result of great physical or mental effort[78] or overwork[84]. This essence is also indicated for periods of convalescence and stress[12]. The indication for White Chestnut flower is for individuals who suffer from excessive thoughts or cyclical thoughts, mental debates and dialogues, undesirable, worrying, fixed, obsessive thoughts that seem impossible to control[85].

Dr Bach called the Star of Bethlehem essence "the comforter and reliever of pain and sorrow". It is indicated for all the consequences of traumatic experiences, whether physical, mental or spiritual, and states of inner numbness caused by shock, loss or bereavement, as well as treating psychosomatic conditions[48,78].

Walnut is the right remedy to provide constancy and protect the individual from unwanted external influences[47]. This essence is also suitable for people who are hypersensitive to ideas, atmospheres and influences, and who may be temporarily affected by the personality or problems of others, which can affect their interpersonal relationships[44]. For these reasons, Walnut is useful for therapists, healthcare workers and professionals who deal with clients who are emotionally disturbed or who may exhaust them emotionally. Intervention Group (IG): received a formula consisting of two drops each of the following essences: Cherry Plum, Elm, Hornbeam, Olive, Star of Bethlehem, Walnut and White Chestnut, produced and manufactured by Bach Flower Remedies Ltd.®, diluted in a vehicle consisting of mineral water and 30 per cent brandy.Placebo group (GP): received an inert vehicle made up of mineral water and 30% brandy, with the same appearance and flavour as GI. The GP and GI bottles were prepared by the researcher. The amber glass dropper bottles had a 75mm glass cannula, perforated cap, black seal and bulb, which had been previously sanitised and sterilised by boiling and heat. The vials were packaged in a brown polybag envelope to keep them safe and intact during transport, and labelled with the participant's name, category, and the name of the participant. professional, work shift and workplace. All the bottles were labelled "treatment bottle" (Figure 1).

Figure 1: Labelled polybag envelope and amber glass bottle with dropper.

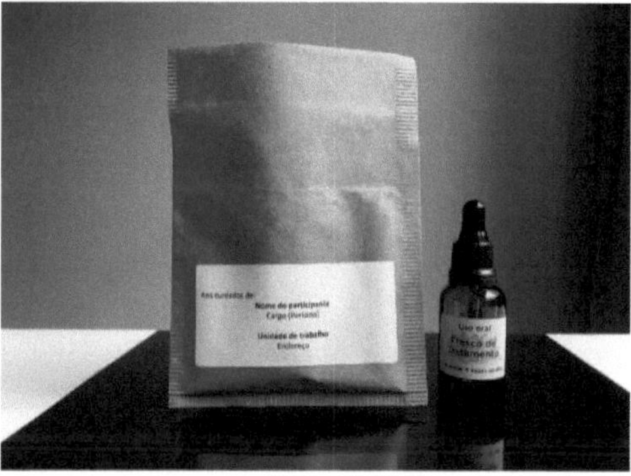

The indicated dosage was four drops, four times a day, every day, distributed as follows: on waking, in the late morning, in the late afternoon and before bed, directly into the mouth. The duration of use was four weeks.

Other guidelines for using the formula included: keeping the bottles away from electronic devices; storing them in a dry, cool and ventilated place, away from humidity and heat; avoiding contamination of the dropper tip and keeping the glass tightly closed after use.

Outcomes, study variables and collection instruments

The primary outcome was assessed by analysing the Perceived Stress Scale and the secondary outcomes were assessed by analysing the Brunel Mood Scale and self-perceived psycho-emotional state. The Perceived Stress Scale (PSS-14) is an adaptation of the Perceived Stress Scale, which measures the degree to which individuals perceive situations in their lives as unpredictable, uncontrollable and overwhelming (Appendix 1). The instrument was validated for Brazilian Portuguese and its psychometric characteristics met the criteria for internal consistency (Cronbach's alpha of 0.82) and construct validity (exploratory factor analysis with orthogonal rotation using the varimax method), making it valid for measuring perceived stress in multicultural studies. As it does not contain context-specific questions, the PSS-14 can be applied to different age groups to measure stress[86].

The scale is made up of 14 questions on a likert scale, the answers to which range from 0 to 4, where 0 = never, 1 = almost never, 2 = sometimes, 3 = almost always and 4 = always[87]. The positive questions (numbers 4, 5, 6, 7, 9, 10 and 13) have their scores added up in reverse[86]. The sum of the scores ranges from zero to 56 points, and can be analysed categorically with five score ranges: < 18 = low stress; 19-24 = normal stress; 25-29 = moderate stress; 30-35 = high stress and > 35 = very high stress. The categorisation of scores does not exist in the original version of the scale, but was suggested by a later study which carried out a confirmatory factor analysis of the three existing versions of the PSS. According to this study, the 5th and 95th percentiles show the extremes of stress proportionality and the 50th percentile characterised the average parameter, stratifying the score into 5 levels: 25th percentile = low; 50th percentile = normal; 75th percentile = moderate; 90th percentile = high; 95th percentile = very high[88].

Mood is considered a relevant indicator of psychological well-being[89]. The Brunel Mood Scale - BRUMS (Appendix 2) is made up of 24 questions divided into six domains, namely Confusion (dazedness, instability in controlling emotions and attention), Depression (emotional isolation, sadness, difficulty adapting, negative self-image), Fatigue (exhaustion, apathy and low level of energy). energy), Anger (hostility and antipathy towards others and oneself), Tension (musculoskeletal) and Vigour (disposition and physical energy)[90]. The answers are coded on a Likert scale ranging from 0 = not at all, 1 = a little, 2 = moderately, 3 = a lot, 4 = extremely. The instrument was validated for Portuguese and the results indicate a good performance in the validation criteria with high values for explained variance, factor loadings and Cronbach's alpha (above 0.70 for all domains), and it was considered an appropriate instrument for assessing mood profiles[91]. This instrument is analysed by assessing the six domains individually. The value for each domain ranges from 0 to 16. Self-perception of the psycho-emotional state was obtained using the Free Word Recall (FWR) technique. The ELP has its origins in Aristotle's Associationist Theory of Memorisation, and was used in the context of clinical psychology by Carl Jung in 1905[92]. The purpose of the ELP was to access the emotional states of the participants before and after the intervention, to see if there were any differences in the words of the Central Nucleus between the study groups.

The professionals were asked to write down the first five words that came to mind to the question "How are you feeling at the moment?", organising the answers in order of importance, from the most important - 1 to the least important - 5[93].

The primary and secondary outcome variables were collected in the at the beginning and end of the intervention. Coping (coping strategies), spiritual well-being and self-reported spirituality were considered moderating variables.

Coping was obtained using the Brief Cope[94], a reduced version of the COPE inventory that assesses the strategies used by individuals in stressful situations (Appendix 3). The instrument has been validated for Brazilian Portuguese and has adequate psychometric properties for its application It has a good Cronbach's alpha of 0.84[95] and can be used to assess coping in stressful situations. It consists of 28 items distributed in 14 dimensions with two items each. The answers are given on a Likert scale ranging from 1 to 4, where 1 = I haven't done it at all, 2 = I've done it a little, 3 = I've done it more or less, to 4 = I've done it a lot[95]. The final score is calculated as the average of the two items corresponding to each dimension, with higher scores corresponding to greater use of a given coping strategy[94].

Spiritual Well-being was measured using the Spiritual Well-being Scale (SWS), one of the pioneering scales on the subject, developed in 1982 by Paloutzian and Ellison (Appendix 4). It has been validated for Brazilian Portuguese and the analyses carried out indicate that the scale has excellent psychometric properties, that it measures the construct it is intended to measure, and has excellent internal consistency measured by Cronbach's alpha of 0.92[96]. This instrument has 20 items divided into two sub-scales: Religious Well-being - BER (measures personal satisfaction with God) and Existential Well-being - BEE (evaluates the existence of a purpose in life independent of religion), both with 10 questions[35]. The answers are presented on a 6-point scale ranging from 1 to 6, with Totally Disagree (TD) = 1, Disagree more than Agree (DC) = 2, Partially Disagree (PD) = 3; Partially Agree (CP) = 4; Agree more than Disagree (CD) = 5, Totally Agree (TC) = 6 for the positive questions (numbers 3, 4, 7, 8, 10, 11, 14, 15, 17, 19 and 20), and this score is inverted for the negative questions[96]. The sum of the scores ranges from 20 to 120, and the cut-off point suggested by the authors who developed the scale is: 20 to 40 = low spiritual well-being; 41 to 99 = moderate spiritual well-being and 100 to 120 = high spiritual well-being[32].

Self-reported spirituality: obtained using a visual numerical scale scored from zero (not at all spiritualised) to 10 (extremely spiritualised). spiritualised), based on the definition of spirituality adopted in the study. The conceptual premise of spirituality in this study defined it as "an individual's propensity or set of beliefs that seeks meaning in life. This meaning for life is sought through a relationship with the transcendent (something beyond the material, earthly plane)" and/or "a sense of connection with something greater than oneself, which transmits vigour, energy and meaning to life events, whether these events are good or bad". It's important to emphasise that spirituality may or may not be linked to the sacred and religion.The moderating variables were only collected at the beginning of the intervention. To characterise the population, an instrument was used with information to obtain the following variables:

•Gender at birth: dichotomous variable (female, male).

•Age: continuous quantitative variable (in years).

•Marital status: nominal variable categorised as single, married or in a stable union, separated or divorced, and widowed.

•Children: dichotomous variable (yes or no).

•Number of children: discrete quantitative variable.

•Education: ordinal variable (primary school, secondary school, higher education, lato sensu - further training / specialisation / residency, master's degree and doctorate).

•Professional category: nominal variable (nurse, nursing technician, nursing assistant).

•Working in the Family Health Strategy (ESF): dichotomous variable (yes and no).

•Work shift: nominally variable (morning, afternoon, full-time).

•Time since graduating in nursing: continuous quantitative variable (in years).

•Time of time in nursing: continuous continuous quantitative variable (in years).

•Number of jobs: discrete quantitative variable.

•Frequency of cigarette consumption: ordinal variable (daily, a few times a week, socially, ex-smoker, never).

•Frequency of drinking alcohol: ordinal variable (daily, a few times a week, socially, never).

•Health problem in drug treatment: dichotomous variable (yes and no).

•Type of medication: nominal variable (according to reports).

•Treatment with mental health professionals: nominal variable (no treatment, treatment with psychologist, treatment with psychiatrist, treatment with psychologist and psychiatrist).

•Number of hours of sleep: continuous quantitative variable (in hours).

•Perceived quality of sleep: ordinal variable (great, good, regular, bad/sleep disorders).

•Use of integrative and complementary practice (ICP): dichotomous variable (yes and no).

• Type of PICS nominal variable (according to reports).

• Previous use of flower therapy: dichotomous variable (yes and no).

The variables for characterising the population were only collected at the start of the intervention.

Treatment-related variables included:

• Expectation of treatment: ordinal nominal variable (complete improvement, moderate improvement, slight improvement, no improvement and can't say). The variable was obtained through the question: "With regard to stress and mood, what do you expect the results to be with the use of the treatment bottle?". Variable collected at the beginning of the intervention.

• Adherence to treatment: obtained by the frequency of use of the formula as directed (four drops, four times a day). Ordinal variable (5 to 7 times a week; 3 to 4 times a week; 1 to 2 times a week; and I took it only when I remembered). Variable collected at the end of the intervention.

• Perception of the study group: dichotomous nominal variable (PG and IG). Variable collected at the end of the intervention.

• Perception of change attributed to treatment: dichotomous nominal variable (yes or no). Variable collected at the end of the intervention.

Data collection

All the data collection procedures were adapted to the research during the COVID-19 pandemic. The invitation to take part in the research was sent by the nursing coordinators of the municipality of Osasco to PHC nursing professionals via the WhatsApp application in the work group. This message included an explanatory video about the project and a link to the electronic Intention to Participate form to be filled in by those interested. This electronic form contained contact details and questions about the eligibility criteria. As the desired number of participants for the study was not reached at this time, a new recruitment process was carried out at the CSEGPS. The researcher was invited by the nurse in charge of the unit to attend a team meeting and explain the objectives of the research to the professionals. At this meeting, leaflets were distributed containing the QR code to access the electronic Intention to Participate form. Eligible participants received the initial electronic form containing the biosociodemographic instrument, the EEP-14 and BRUMS scales, Brief Cope and EBE, and questions regarding self-reported spirituality, self-perceived psycho-emotional state (PEMS) and expectation of outcome with the treatment bottle. According to the randomised list, participants were allocated to either the GP or the IG. The bottles were mostly delivered by a delivery service to the workplace and a few deliveries were made by the researcher. Instructions for use were sent via WhatsApp. The researcher contacted the participants via WhatsApp on a weekly basis to answer questions, check on their adaptation to the treatment and any needs they might have, such as the supply of a new bottle due to breakage or loss. After four weeks, the participants were instructed to fill in the electronic Closure form, containing the EEP-14 and BRUMS instruments, and the questions on psycho-emotional self-perception (ELP), adherence to the use of the bottle received, new health treatments started, perception of the treatment group they were in and perception of changes that occurred with the use of the bottle. At the end of the research, all the participants received a report containing their results and a bottle of the flower formula to ensure continuity of treatment. Figure 2 summarises the collection forms and instruments according to when they were completed.

Figure 2: Electronic forms and the instruments they contain.

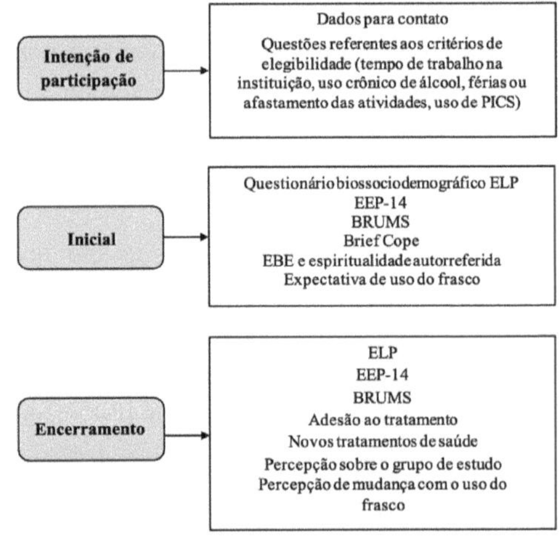

Analysing the data

Descriptive measures of absolute and relative frequencies, central tendency and variability were used to characterise the population. To compare the homogeneity of the groups, the Chi-square or Fisher's Exact tests were used for the qualitative variables and the Student's t-test or Wilcoxon-Mann-Whitney test for the quantitative variables, according to the normality of the data. The normality of the data was checked using quantile-quantile diagrams (Q-Q diagrams).Linear mixed model (LMM) analysis by time and group was used to evaluate the intervention. This type of analysis offers more flexibility than repeated measures ANOVA, uses all available data, is not affected by missing data and can flexibly model the effects of time[97]. The effect size (TDE) was measured by the Eta square (η^2) partial, and presented according to the classification: 0.0099 - small TDE; 0.0588 - medium TDE; 0.1379 - large TDE[98]. The significance level adopted was 5%. The analysis was carried out by a statistician using the $R^{®}$ package version 4.2.2.

Prototypical analysis, a technique used in the study of social representations, was used to assess the ELP. In prototypical analysis, the elements that are most important to the individual are more accessible to their consciousness[99]. The technique consists of combining the frequency and Average Order of Recall (OME) of words to create a four-quadrant table representing the elements that are central to the group under study[100]. After correcting the spelling, the words evoked were lemmatised to avoid similar words being considered different. For example, the terms "anxious", "anxious" and "anxiety" were grouped together in the "anxious" category, which was the term that appeared most frequently. Each corpus was then submitted to the free online software openEvoc 0.94, which compiled a list of the words evoked in alphabetical order for each one, calculated the total frequency, the frequency of evocation in each position and the OME, and organised the evocations in four-quadrant tables[101].

OME takes into account the position in which the word was evoked by the individual and its frequency[102-104]. In this study, the average order of importance was used as the OME, since the hierarchisation of the terms was carried out by the participant themselves. For illustration purposes, here is an example of the calculation of the OME of the term "Anxious", from the GP, before the intervention:

Category = Anxious	
Number of times it was mentioned and ranked in 1st place	8
Number of times it was mentioned and ranked in 2nd place	4
Number of times it was mentioned and ranked in 3rd place	3
Number of times it was mentioned and ranked in 4th place	3
Number of times it was mentioned and ranked in 5th place	1
Total frequency	19
OME = [(8x1)+(4x2)+(3x3)+(3x4)+(1x5)] / 19	2,21

Establishing the OME cut-off point for drawing up the table depends on the number of words the participants are asked to recall. In studies that ask participants to recall an even number of words, the average OME of the words included in the analysis is calculated. If an odd number of words are requested, the cut-off point used is the median[100,104]. In this study, participants were asked to recall five words, so the OME cut-off point is three. The OME indicates the degree of importance of each word, and its values ranged from 1.0 to 5.0, with values close to 1.0 being more relevant and values closer to 5.0 being less relevant[103].

The minimum frequency for a term to be included in the analysis was calculated by dividing the total frequency of evocations by the number of different evocations [total frequency of evocations / number of different evocations][100]. With regard to the frequency cut-off point, in this study we used half the frequency of the evocation with the highest occurrence in the corpus. For example, if the word with the highest frequency had 16 evocations, the cut-off point was eight[104]. Once the cut-off points had been defined, the software built the four-quadrant tables. The first quadrant is made up o f elements of the Central Core (frequency $\geq$ average frequency and OME < average evocation OME). The second quadrant is the First Periphery (frequency $\geq$ average frequency and OME $\geq$ average OME). The third quadrant is the Contrast Zone (frequency < average frequency and OME < average recall OME). In the fourth quadrant (frequency < average frequency and OME $\geq$ average recall OME) is observed a Second Periphery[104-105]. To assess the self-perception of the psycho-emotional state, the evocations of the Central Nucleus quadrant were analysed.

Chart 1: Example of the construction of a four-quadrant board.

Central Centre	First Periphery
Frequency ≥ average frequency and OME < average recall OME Readily evoked and frequent terms	Frequency ≥ average frequency and OME ≥ average recall OME Late and frequent terms
Contrast Zone	Second Periphery
Frequency < average frequency and OME < average recall OME Readily evoked and infrequent terms	Frequency < average frequency and OME ≥ average recall OME Late and infrequent terms

All the procedures were repeated for the two study groups separately, before and after the intervention. To analyse the ELP, only the data from the participants who completed the study were taken into account.

Ethical aspects

The project was authorised by the co-participating institutions and approved by the Research Ethics Committees of the USP School of Nursing with opinion no. 4.804.586 and the USP School of Public Health with opinion no. 5.489.450. It was carried out in accordance with Resolution 466/2012, the guidelines of the National Research Ethics Council (CONEP) for data collection in a virtual environment and the General Data Protection Law 13.709/2018. By clicking on the link to access the initial electronic form, the participants were automatically directed to the Informed Consent Form (ICF) page, with all the information about the study and the communication channel with the researcher, in this case the e-form. e-mail and the address of the study's website. After reading the ICF, the participant chose one of three options: A) I agree to voluntarily participate in the research; B) I do not agree to participate in the research; C) I have questions about the research and would like clarification before agreeing to participate. The instrument could only be accessed if the participant chose the option A. If they chose option B, they were directed to a thank-you page and their participation was terminated. If they chose option C, they had access to a field to describe their doubts, which were answered by the researcher. This strategy was necessary to guarantee freedom of participation in the research and access to the instruments only after agreeing to the ICF. The link to the printable version was available at the end of the TCLE text and on the home page of the study website. All personal data was anonymised. In order to guarantee the security of the information and reduce the possibility of undue access, all forms were removed from the virtual environment after the collection was completed. The study was approved and published in the Brazilian Registry of Clinical Trials (ReBEC) under the code RBR-4wzz4xy.

RESULTS

A total of 113 nursing professionals filled in the electronic Intention to Participate form. Of these, 26 didn't take part in the study, two because they didn't meet the inclusion criteria (they were away on sick leave) and 24 because they gave up before completing the initial electronic form, resulting in a sample of 87 participants randomised between the groups: 44 (51%) in the GP and 43 (49%) in the IG (Figure 3). No participant had self-reported alcoholism, previous use of flower therapy or use of PICS during the study.

Figure 3: Flowchart of the clinical trial. São Paulo, Brazil, 2022

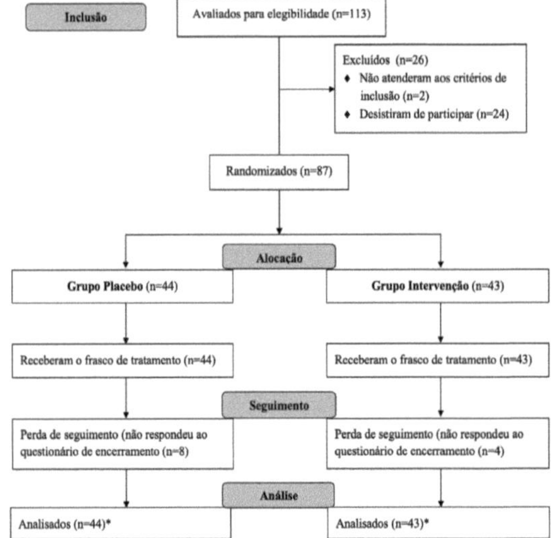

* The statistical analysis used allowed for the inclusion of individuals who did not finalise the survey.

No harm was reported during the study. Only one participant in the GP reported drowsiness when using the formula and dropped out of the study.

Biosociodemographic and professional characterisation of the population

The sample was made up of 92% women (n=80), with an average age of 44.7 (±9.3) years, 57.5% married or in a stable union, with an average of 1.6 (±1.2) children. With regard to professional category, 70.2 per cent of the participants were technical professionals (n=61), with an average of 1.3 (±0.5) jobs, 14.8 (±8.0) years of training and 8.3 (±7.7) years working in nursing. Of the technical professionals, 21.3% (n=13) had a university degree and 9.8% (n=6) had a specialisation or residency. Among the nurses, 76.9% (n=20) had a specialisation or residency. The distribution of sociodemographic variables by study group is shown in Table 1. The groups were homogeneous for all variables.

Table 1: Distribution of participants according to sociodemographic variables, by study group. São Paulo, Brazil, 2022.

			GP	GI		
Variable	Categories	N	%	N	%	p-value
Age group	23 - 30	-	-	3	7,0	0,154*
	31 - 40	14	31,8	13	30,2	
	41 - 50	15	34,1	20	46,5	
	51 - 60	11	25,0	6	14,0	
	61 - 68	4	9,1	1	2,3	
Sex	Female	41	93,2	39	90,7	0,672**
	Male	3	6,8	4	9,3	
Marital status	Single	7	15,9	13	30,2	0,178*
	Married/Stable Union	27	61,4	23	53,5	
	Divorced	7	15,9	7	16,3	
	Widowed	3	6,8	-	-	
No. of children	0	8	18,2	10	23,3	0,973*
	1	13	29,5	14	32,5	
	2	13	29,5	11	25,5	
	3	6	13,6	6	14,0	
	4	3	6,9	2	4,7	
	5	1	2,3	-	-	
Education	Medium	20	45,4	23	53,5	0,611**
	Superior	12	27,3	8	18,6	
	Lato Sensu	12	27,3	12	27,9	
Category professional	Auxiliary	5	11,3	2	4,6	0,150**
	Technical	23	52,3	31	72,1	
	Nurse	16	36,4	10	23,3	
Time of training in nursing	< 1 - 5 years	5	11,4	10	23,3	0.245**
	6 - 0 years	6	13,6	5	11,6	
	11 - 15 years	15	34,0	7	16,3	
	16 - 20 years	9	20,5	13	30,2	
	21 - 32 years old	9	20,5	8	18,6	
Time of work at	< 1 - 5 years	25	56,8	21	48,8	0,818*
	6 - 10 years	3	6,8	2	4,7	

nursing	11 - 15 years	8	18,2	12	27,8	
	16 - 20 years	5	11,4	6	14,0	
	21 - 37 years***	3	6,8	2	4,7	
ESF	No	34	77,3	34	79,1	0,840**
	Yes	10	22,7	9	20,9	
Shift	Integral	11	25,0	13	30,2	0,621**
	Morning	22	50,0	17	39,6	
	Afternoon	11	25,0	13	30,2	
Links	1	32	72,7	30	69,0	0,945**
employment	2 or 3	12	27,3	13#	31,0	

* Fisher's Exact Test. ** Chi-squared test. *** Participant probably started in nursing as an assistant, given that the maximum training time in nursing was 32 years. # A professional with 3 jobs. GP = placebo group. IG = intervention group. ESF = Family Health Strategy.

Table 2 shows the participants according to habits and health problems by study group. The most prevalent health problems undergoing drug treatment among the participants were systemic arterial hypertension - SAH (n=20; 23%); depression (n=9; 10.3%) and diabetes mellitus - DM (n=8; 9.2%). With regard to mental health treatment, 11.5% (n=10) of the participants were being monitored by a psychologist, 4.6% (n=4) by a psychiatrist and 4.6% (n=4) by both a psychologist and a psychiatrist. Participants' sleep was also assessed in the study, with an average of 6.3 (±1.3) hours of sleep per night and most of the quality reported as regular (n=48; 55.2%).

Table 2: Distribution of participants according to habits and health problems in treatment, by study group. São Paulo, Brazil, 2022.

Variable	Categories	GP		GI		
		N	%	N	%	p-value
Cigarette use	Sometimes in the week	-	-	2	4,7	
	Daily	5	11,4	4	9,3	0,247*
	Ex-smoker	2	4,5	3	7,0	
	Never	37	84,1	31	72,0	
	Socially	-	-	3	7,0	
Alcohol use	Sometimes in the week	1	2,3	2	4,7	0,657**
	Never	20	45,4	16	37,2	
	Socially	23	52,3	25	58,1	
Hypertension	No	32	72,7	35	81,4	0,339*

							*
arterial	Yes	12	27,3	8		18,6	
Depression	No	39	88,6	39		90,7	0,479**
	Yes	5	11,4	4		9,3	
Diabetes	No	39	88,6	40		93,0	0,481**
	Yes	5	11,4	3		7,0	
Disorders	No	41	93,1	40		93,0	0,977**
thyroid	Yes	3	6,9	3		7,0	
Obesity	No	44	100,0	42		97,7	0,494*
	Yes	-	-	1		2,3	
Chronic pain	No	42	95,5	42		97,7	0,573**
	Yes	2	4,5	1		2,3	
Migraine	No	42	95,5	42		97,7	0,573**
	Yes	2	4,5	1		2,3	
Contraceptive	No	42	95,5	42		97,7	0,573**
oral	Yes	2	4,5	1		2,3	
Dyslipidaemia	No	42	95,5	41		95,3	0,981**
	Yes	2	4,5	2		4,7	
Dermatitis	No	44	100,0	42		97,7	0,494*
atopic	Yes	0	-	1		2,3	
Glaucoma	No	44	100,0	42		97,7	0,494*
	Yes	0	-	1		2,3	
Anxiety	No	41	93,2	41		95,4	0,666**
	Yes	3	6,8	2		4,6	

* Fisher's Exact Test. ** Chi-squared test. GP = placebo group. IG = intervention group. The groups were homogeneous for all clinical and health variables, except for sleep quality (p = 0.004), in which the GP had better sleep quality compared to the GI.

Expectations and adherence to treatment

Participants were asked at the start of the study about their expectations of the treatment in terms of stress and mood levels, and 13 participants (14.9%) expected a slight improvement, 35 (40.3%) a slight improvement and 10 (40.3%) a slight improvement. moderate improvement, 13 (14.9%) a complete improvement and 26 (29.9%) didn't know what to expect from the treatment. No participant expected any improvement from using the bottle.

At the end of the study, the participants answered questions about using the bottle as directed, their perception of the group in which they took part and their perception of change with the use of the formula. With regard to using the bottle, eight participants (10.7%) took it as directed less than twice a week, 34 (45.3%) three to four times a week and 33 (44.0%) five to seven times a week. With regard to the perception of the study group, 48 participants (64.0%) believed they were in the IG, 22 (29.3%) in the PG and five (6.7%) couldn't say. When asked about perceived changes with the treatment, 47 participants (62.7%) perceived changes in stress and mood and 28 (37.3%) said they did not perceive any changes. The groups were also homogeneous for these variables (Table 3).

Table 3: Participants' expectations regarding the result of using the bottle, frequency of bottle use according to indication, perception of study group and perception of change, by study group. São Paulo, Brazil, 2022.

		GP		GI			
Variable	Categories	N	%	N	%	p-value	
Expectations	I can't say	13	29,5	13	30,2	0,452*	
regarding	No improvement	-	-	-	-		
bottle use	Slight improvement	9	20,5	4	9,3		
	Moderately	17	38,6	18	41,9		
	Completely	5	11,4	8	18,6		
Use of the bottle	Less than 2 times/week	5	13,9	3	7,7	0,505**	
according to	3 to 4 times/week	14	38,9	20	51,3		
indication	5 to 7 times/week	17	47,2	16	41,0		
Perception	GP	14	38,8	8	20,5	0,209**	
group	GI	20	55,6	28	71,8		
study	I don't know	2	5,6	3	7,7		
Perception of	Yes	19	52,8	28	71,8	0,089*	
change	No	17	47,2	11	28,2		

* Chi-squared test. ** Fisher's Exact Test. GP = placebo group. IG = intervention group.

Characterisation of the population in terms of moderating variables

The type of coping most used by the participants was Problem-Focused Coping and the most used strategies were Planning, followed by Religion and Positive Reinterpretation.The two study groups were homogeneous in terms of coping strategies and types, except for the Denial strategy, which was used more by GI (Table 4).

Table 4: Distribution of values for the dimensions and types of coping in the scale Brief Cope by study group, before the intervention. São Paulo, Brazil, 2022.

Variables	Group	N	Average	DP	Median	Min	Max	p-value
Self-blame	GP	44	2,6	1,0	2,5	1,0	4,0	0,997*
	GI	43	2,6	0,9	2,5	1,0	4,0	
Abuse of	GP	44	1,3	0,6	1,0	1,0	3,0	0,473*
substances	GI	43	1,4	0,7	1,0	1,0	4,0	
Denial	GP	44	2,1	0,9	2,0	1,0	4,0	0,025*
	GI	43	2,5	0,9	2,5	1,0	4,0	
Divestment	GP	44	1,9	1,0	1,5	1,0	4,0	0,895*
behavioural	GI	43	1,8	0,8	1,5	1,0	4,0	
Self-distraction	GP	44	2,7	0,8	2,5	1,0	4,0	0,598*
	GI	43	2,6	0,7	2,5	1,0	4,0	
Humour	GP	44	1,7	0,7	1,5	1,0	3,5	0,768*
	GI	43	1,7	0,9	1,5	1,0	4,0	
Spirituality	GP	44	2,2	0,8	2,0	1,0	4,0	0,405*
	GI	43	2,4	0,8	2,0	1,0	4,0	
Religion	GP	44	2,9	1,1	3,0	1,0	4,0	0,614*
	GI	43	3,1	1,0	3,0	1,0	4,0	
Active coping	GP	44	2,8	0,8	2,5	1,0	4,0	0,534*
	GI	43	2,9	0,8	3,0	1,0	4,0	
Planning	GP	44	2,9	0,7	3,0	1,0	4,0	0,367*
	GI	43	3,1	0,8	3,0	1,5	4,0	
Reinterpreta tion	GP	44	2,8	0,9	3,0	1,0	4,0	0,795*
positive	GI	43	2,9	0,8	3,0	1,5	4,0	
Acceptance	GP	44	2,9	0,8	3,0	1,0	4,0	0,084**
	GI	43	2,6	0,8	2,5	1,0	4,0	
Support	GP	44	2,4	1,0	2,5	1,0	4,0	0,860*
instrumental	GI	43	2,5	1,0	2,5	1,0	4,0	
Support	GP	44	2,3	1,1	2,0	1,0	4,0	0,897*
emotional	GI	43	2,3	1,0	2,5	1,0	4,0	
Focussed	GP	44	2,7	0,6	2,7	1,7	3,9	0,938**
problem	GI	43	2,7	0,7	2,8	1,6	4,0	
Focussed	GP	44	2,4	0,5	2,4	1,4	3,5	0,695**
Functional emotion	GI	43	2,4	0,5	2,5	1,0	4,0	
Focussed	GP	44	2,0	0,6	1,8	1,0	3,5	0,299**
dysfunction al emotion	GI	43	2,1	0,5	2,1	1,0	3,3	

* Wilcoxon-Mann-Whitney test. ** Student's t-test. PG = placebo group. IG = intervention group.

Cronbach's alpha reliability was 0.805 for Brief Cope, 0.841 for Problem-Focused Coping, 0.609 for Functional Emotion-Focused Coping and 0.701 for Dysfunctional Emotion-Focused Coping. The mean EBE score in this study was 92.2 (±20.0), which classifies the level of spiritual well-being as moderate. The average self-reported spirituality score was 7.9 (±1.8).

The study groups were homogeneous for spiritual well-being and its dimensions, and for self-reported spirituality (Table 5).

Table 5: Distribution of the values of the EBE scale and its dimensions and self-reported spirituality, by study group, before the intervention. São Paulo, Brazil, 2022.

Variable	Group	N	Average	DP	Median	Minimum	Maximum	p-value*
BEE	GP	44	42,9	10,8	44,0	15,0	59,0	0,233
	GI	43	41,4	8,3	41,0	20,0	57,0	
BER	GP	44	49,3	13,7	54,5	10,0	60,0	0,648
	GI	43	50,9	10,8	56,0	20,0	60,0	
EBE	GP	44	92,2	22,4	100,0	25,0	119,0	0,538
	GI	43	92,3	17,5	97,0	49,0	117,0	
Spirit. autoref	GP	44	7,9	2,0	8,0	2,0	10,0	0,851
	GI	43	8,0	1,6	8,0	5,0	10,0	

* Wilcoxon-Mann-Whitney test

BEE = existential well-being; BER = religious well-being; EBE = spiritual well-being scale; Esp self-ref = self-reported spirituality. PG = placebo group. IG = intervention group. SD = standard deviation

Cronbach's alpha reliability was 0.927 for the EBE, 0.943 for the BEE domain and 0.826 for the BER domain.

Characterisation of the population in terms of primary and secondary outcome variables

The study groups were homogeneous in terms of stress levels before the intervention (Table 6) and began the study with an average perceived stress of 31.1 (±8.2), classified as high stress.

Table 6: Distribution of the values of the perceived stress variable, by study group, before the intervention. São Paulo, Brazil, 2022.

Variable Group N Mean MPD Median Minimum Maximum p-value*

Variable	Group	N	Mean	MPD	Median	Minimum	Maximum	p-value*
Stress	GP	44	30,4	8,9	28,0	8,0	50,0	0,485
realised	GI	43	31,7	7,5	31,0	16,0	45,0	

* Student's t-test.

GP = placebo group. IG = intervention group. SD = standard deviation

Cronbach's alpha reliability was 0.910 for the EEP-14. The groups were also homogeneous in terms of mood levels and their dimensions, except for Vigour, where the GP had higher values than the GI (Table 7). The BRUMS dimensions with the highest means were Fatigue (9.8±3.9), followed by Tension (7.7±3.3).

Table 7: Distribution of mood domain values, by study group, before the intervention. São Paulo, Brazil, 2022.

Variable	Group	N	Average	DP	Median	Minimum	Maximum	p-value
Depression	GP	44	6,6	4,0	6,0	0,0	16,0	0,676*
	GI	43	7,0	3,6	7,0	0,0	13,0	
Confusion	GP	44	4,8	3,2	4,5	0,0	14,0	0,513**
	GI	43	5,2	2,9	5,0	0,0	13,0	
Fatigue	GP	44	9,6	4,2	10,5	1,0	16,0	0,868**
	GI	43	9,9	3,7	10,0	2,0	16,0	
Anger	GP	44	5,6	4,3	4,5	0,0	16,0	0,474**
	GI	43	6,1	4,0	5,0	0,0	16,0	
Tension	GP	44	7,7	3,3	8,0	1,0	16,0	0,956*
	GI	43	7,7	3,4	8,0	2,0	15,0	
Vigour	GP	44	6,4	3,1	6,5	1,0	13,0	0,038*
	GI	43	5,2	2,6	5,0	1,0	11,0	

* Student's t-test; ** Wilcoxon-Mann-Whitney test

GP = placebo group. IG = intervention group. SD = standard deviation

Cronbach's alpha reliability was 0.914 for BRUMS, 0.882 for the Depression domain, 0.786 for Confusion, 0.861 for Fatigue, 0.906 for Anger, 0.807 for Tension and 0.751 for Vigour.

Analysing the outcome of the intervention and interactions

When analysing the effect of the intervention, it was found that there was no significant difference between the groups over the course of the study. Both the PG and IG showed a reduction in the scores of the PDE-14, Global Mood and negative dimensions of the BRUMS, and an increase in the Vigour dimension. Figure 3 illustrates how the scores of the outcome variables behaved over the course of the study.

Figure 3: Comparison of outcome variables according to study groups over the course of the intervention. São Paulo, Brazil, 2022.

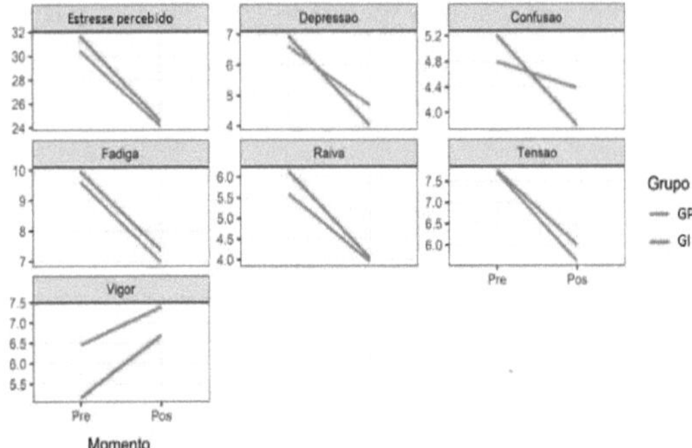

Table 8 shows that there was no significant difference in the levels of perceived stress between the study groups, with the PSS-14 values decreasing and the classification going from high stress to normal stress in both groups at the end of the intervention. However, there was a statistically significant reduction in the values of this intra-group variable.

Table 8: Mean, standard deviation, confidence interval and p-value of the perceived stress variable in the study groups. São Paulo, Brazil, 2022.

Variable	Group	Moment	N	Average	DP	p-value 95%CI moment1	p-value group: Moment2
Stress	GP	Pre	44	30,4	8,9	[27,9; 33,1]	
realised		Post	36	24,1	9,2	[21,4; 27,3] 0,038*	0,750*
	GI	Pre	43	31,7	7,5	[29,4; 33,9]	
		Post	39	24,5	7,9	[21,9; 26,8]	

* LMM. [1] Intra-group. [2] Between groups

GP = placebo group. IG = intervention group. SD = standard deviation. CI = confidence interval.

Table 9 shows that there was no significant difference in the participants' mood levels in any of the domains. Both groups showed a reduction in the Depression, Confusion, Anger, Fatigue and Tension scores and an increase in the Vigour score.

Table 9: Mean, standard deviation, confidence interval and p-value of the mood domains in the study groups. São Paulo, Brazil, 2022.

Variable	Group	Moment	N	Average	DP	95%CI	p-value moment1	p-value group: moment2
Depression	GP	Pre	44	6,6	4,0	[5,5; 7,9]	0,238*	0,993*
		Post	36	4,7	4,6	[3,3; 6,3]		
	GI	Pre	43	7,0	3,6	[5,9; 8,0]		
		Post	39	4,0	3,6	[3,0; 5,2]		
Confusion	GP	Pre	44	4,8	3,2	[3,9; 5,8]	0,350*	0,213*
		Post	36	4,4	3,8	[3,3; 5,8]		
	GI	Pre	43	5,2	2,9	[4,4; 6,1]		
		Post	39	3,8	3,4	[2,8; 5,0]		
Fatigue	GP	Pre	44	9,6	4,2	[8,3; 10,8]	0,366*	0,306*
		Post	36	7,0	4,3	[5,6; 8,4]		
	GI	Pre	43	10,0	3,7	[8,8; 11,0]		
		Post	39	7,4	4,2	[6,1; 8,7]		
Anger	GP	Pre	44	5,6	4,3	[4,4; 7,0]	0,746*	0,937*
		Post	36	3,9	4,5	[2,7; 5,7]		
	GI	Pre	43	6,1	4,0	[5,0; 7,4]		
		Post	39	4,0	3,6	[3,0; 5,3]		
Tension	GP	Pre	44	7,7	3,3	[6,8; 8,7]	0,131*	0,320*
		Post	36	5,6	3,5	[4,6; 6,8]		
	GI	Pre	43	7,7	3,4	[6,8; 8,8]		
		Post	39	6,0	3,7	[4,9; 7,1]		
Vigour	GP	Pre	44	6,5	3,1	[5,6; 7,4]	0,249*	0,850*
		Post	36	7,4	3,6	[6,2; 8,5]		
	GI	Pre	43	5,2	2,6	[4,4; 6,0]		
		Post	39	6,7	2,5	[5,9; 7,5]		

* LMM. [1] Intra-group. [2] Between groups

GP = placebo group. IG = intervention group. SD = standard deviation. CI = confidence interval.

In addition to evaluating the outcomes of the intervention, some interactions were also tested. The aim of these regression models was to assess the percentage that the moderating variables and some sociodemographic and health variables influenced the results found in the outcomes.The first regression model tested the interaction of the outcomes with the variables Denial coping, Acceptance coping and the BEE domain of the EBE, sleep quality and marital status.

Table 10 shows that timing, the BEE variable (p<0.001), the Moment:Acceptance interaction (p=0.007) and sleep quality (p=0.035) influenced participants' perceived stress. Momentum was responsible for 5.7 per cent, BEE for 24.7 per cent, sleep quality for 13.1 per cent, and the Momentum:Acceptance interaction for 5.8 per cent of the variability in this outcome. The BEE variable had a large TDE, the sleep quality and Moment:Acceptance interaction variables had a medium TDE and moment had a small TDE.

Table 10: p-values and effect size of the interaction analyses of the perceived stress outcome. São Paulo, Brazil, 2022.

Variables	p-value*	η2 partial
Moment	0,038	0,057
Group	0,562	0,004
Denial	0,099	0,032
Acceptance	0,513	0,006
BEE	< 0,001	0,247
Sleep quality	0,007	0,131
Marital status	0,551	0,005
Moment:Group	0,750	0,001
Moment:Denial	0,877	0,000
Moment: Acceptance	0,035	0,058
Moment:BEE	0,825	0,001
Moment:Sleep quality	0,299	0,048
Moment:Marital status	0,999	0,000

* LMM. BEE = existential well-being

The interaction analysis showed that BEE (p<0.001) and sleep quality (p=0.008) influenced the Depression dimension. The former was responsible for 30.1 per cent and the latter for 12.8 per cent of the variability in this domain (Table 11). The variables showed a large SDT for BEE and a medium SDT for sleep quality.

Table 11: p-values and effect sizes from interaction analyses of the outcome Depression. São Paulo, Brazil, 2022.

Variables	p-value*	η2 partial
Moment	0,238	0,019
Group	0,063	0,043
Denial	0,185	0,021
Acceptance	0,818	0,001
BEE	< 0,001	0,301
Sleep quality	0,008	0,128
Marital status	0,292	0,014
Moment:Group	0,993	0,000
Moment:Denial	0,348	0,011
Moment: Acceptance	0,105	0,035
Moment:BEE	0,716	0,002
Moment:Sleep quality	0,133	0,069
Moment:Marital status	0,991	0,000

* LMM. BEE = existential well-being

Tables 12, 13, 14 and 15 show that the BEE variable had an influence on the Confusion (p<0.001), Fatigue (p=0.008), Anger (p<0.001) and Tension (p<0.001) dimensions, and was responsible for 28.6 per cent (TDE = large), 8.6 per cent (TDE = medium), 14.1 per cent (TDE = large) and 16.0 per cent (TDE = large) of the variability in these domains, respectively.

Table 12: p-values and effect size of the interaction analyses of the Confusion outcome. São Paulo, Brazil, 2022.

Variables	p-value*	η2 partial
Moment	0,350	0,012
Group	0,599	0,004
Denial	0,883	0,000
Acceptance	0,116	0,032
BEE	<0,001	0,286
Sleep quality	0,453	0,032
Marital status	0,905	0,000
Moment:Group	0,213	0,021
Moment:Denial	0,974	0,000
Moment: Acceptance	0,894	0,000
Moment:BEE	0,301	0,015
Moment:Sleep quality	0,773	0,015
Moment:Marital status	0,456	0,008

* LMM. BEE = existential well-being

Table 13: p-values and effect size of the interaction analyses of the Fatigue outcome. São Paulo, Brazil, 2022.

Variables	p-value*	η2 partial
Moment	0,366	0,011
Group	0,885	0,000
Denial	0,754	0,001
Acceptance	0,534	0,005
BEE	0,008	0,086
Sleep quality	0,256	0,048
Marital status	0,886	0,000
Moment:Group	0,306	0,014
Moment:Denial	0,055	0,047
Moment: Acceptance	0,920	0,000
Moment:BEE	0,210	0,022
Moment:Sleep quality	0,426	0,037
Moment:Marital status	0,503	0,006

* LMM. BEE = existential well-being

Table 14: p-values and effect size of the interaction analyses of the rabies outcome. São Paulo, Brazil, 2022.

Variables	p-value*	η2 partial
Moment	0,746	0,001
Group	0,474	0,007
Denial	0,636	0,003
Acceptance	0,824	0,001
BEE	<0,001	0,141
Sleep quality	0,185	0,057
Marital status	0,774	0,001
Moment:Group	0,937	0,000
Moment:Denial	0,251	0,017
Moment: Acceptance	0,925	0,000
Moment:BEE	0,610	0,004
Moment:Sleep quality	0,398	0,039
Moment:Marital status	0,523	0,006

* LMM. BEE = existential well-being

Table 15: p-values and effect size of the interaction analyses of the Tension outcome. São Paulo, Brazil, 2022.

Variables	p-value*	η2 partial
Moment	0,131	0,031
Group	0,328	0,013
Denial	0,362	0,010
Acceptance	0,879	0,000
BEE	<0,001	0,160
Sleep quality	0,136	0,066
Marital status	0,452	0,007
Moment:Group	0,320	0,013
Moment:Denial	0,759	0,001
Moment: Acceptance	0,267	0,017
Moment:BEE	0,426	0,009
Moment:Sleep quality	0,388	0,039
Moment:Marital status	0,395	0,010
* LMM. BEE = existential well-being		

As seen in Table 16, the interaction analysis showed that BEE (p<0.001) and sleep quality (p<0.001) influenced the Vigour dimension. BEE accounted for 15.7 per cent and sleep quality 21.9 per cent of the variability in this domain. Both variables had a large TDE.

Table 16: p-values and effect size of the interaction analyses for the Vigour outcome. São Paulo, Brazil, 2022.

Variables	p-value*	η2 partial
Moment	0,249	0,018
Group	0,111	0,031
Denial	0,776	0,001
Acceptance	0,612	0,003
BEE	<0,001	0,157
Sleep quality	<0,001	0,219
Marital status	0,850	0,000
Moment:Group	0,850	0,000
Moment:Denial	0,491	0,006
Moment: Acceptance	0,150	0,028
Moment:BEE	0,672	0,003
Moment:Sleep quality	0,784	0,014
Moment:Marital status	0,653	0,003

* LMM. BEE = existential well-being

The second regression model for interaction analysis included The variables Denial coping, Acceptance coping, the BEE domain of the EBE, dichotomous sleep quality, outcome expectancy, dichotomous use of the formula as indicated and dichotomous treatment of mental health problems were analysed to check their influence on the participants' stress and mood levels. BEE had a significant influence on all the outcomes and was responsible for 21.7 per cent of the variability in perceived stress (p<0.001), 28.2 per cent in Depression (p<0.001), 26.5 per cent in Confusion (p<0.001), 7.1 per cent in Fatigue (p=0.026), 12.9 per cent in Anger (p=0.002), 15.3 per cent in Tension (p<0.001) and 9.6 per cent in Vigour (p=0.009). The SDTs were large for the perceived stress, Depression, Confusion and Tension outcomes, and medium for the Fatigue, Anger and Vigour outcomes. The Moment:Acceptance interaction significantly influenced the perceived stress outcome (p=0.039), accounting for 6.2 per cent of its variability, with an average TDE.The outcome expectation variable influenced the Confusion outcome (p=0.036), accounting for 11.8 per cent of its variability, with a mean TDE. Denial coping, sleep quality, use of formula as indicated and treatment for mental health problems had no significant influence on any of the outcomes (p>0.05).

Free word recall analysis

The number of questionnaires answered before the intervention was 75. One questionnaire was discarded because the participant used the same word in all five evocations.Table 2 summarises the analysis of the question about self-perception of psycho-emotional state by the ELP, according to the study group, before the intervention. There was similarity between the groups in terms of the number of categories analysed, minimum word frequency and point of the OME.

Table 2: Number of questionnaires, total number of evocations, categories analysed and cut-off points for evocations before the intervention. São Paulo, Brazil, 2022.

	GI	GP
No. of questionnaires	39	35
Questionnaires excluded	0	1
Total number of evocations	195	175
Categories analysed	16	16
Minimum frequency	3 words	3 words
Frequency cut-off point	11	12
OME cut-off point	3	3

The composition of the Central Core, Contrast Zone and Peripheries of the study groups before the intervention is shown in Tables 3 and 4. When looking at the components of the Central Core, both the IG and the SG found a prevalence of evocations with a negative connotation, with the terms "Tired" and "Anxious" being the most evoked in both groups. The Contrast Zone was much less expressive in the GP, with only two words and a low frequency.

Table 3: Composition of the Central Core, Contrast Zone and Peripheries of the GI before the intervention. São Paulo, Brazil, 2022.

Central Centre			First Periphery		
Frequency ≥ 11 and OME < 3.0			Frequency ≥ 11 and OME ≥ 3.0		
	Frequency	OME		Frequency	OME
Tired Anxious	21 19	2,2 2,7			
Contrast Zone			Second Periphery		
Frequency < 11 and OME < 3.0			Frequency < 11 and OME ≥ 3.0		

	Frequency	OME		Frequency	OME
Worried Happy	10	2,9	Sleepy	9	3,2
Angry Stressed	9	2,1	Discouraged	7	3,1
Well	7	2,7	Anguished Sad	6	3.2
	6	2,8	Demotivated	6	3.2
	3	1,0	Impatient Hopeful	5	3.2
			Nervous Fearful	4	3.5
				4	3.8
				4	4
				3	4.3

Table 4: Composition of the Central Nucleus, Contrast Zone and Peripheries of the GP before the intervention. São Paulo, Brazil, 2022.

Central Centre			First Periphery		
Frequency ≥ 12 and OME < 3.0			Frequency ≥ 12 and OME ≥ 3.0		
	Frequency	OME		Frequency	OME
Tired Anxious	23	2,2			
Worried	19	2,2			
	12	2,3			
Contrast Zone			Second Periphery		
Frequency < 12 and OME < 3.0			Frequency < 12 and OME ≥ 3.0		
	Frequency	OME		Frequency	OME
Angry Quiet	3	2,0	Sad Sleepy	11	3,6
	3	2,3	Stressed	8	3,6
			Thoughtful	7	3,3
			Confident Happy	6	3,0
			Fearful	6	3,2
			Discouraged	6	4,2
			Hopeful	5	3,0
			Anguished	5	3,6
			Insecure	3	3,3
				3	4,0
				3	4,0

After the intervention, 74 questionnaires were analysed (the questionnaire of the participant who answered all five evocations with the same word was discarded).Table 5 summarises the analysis of the question about self-perception of psycho-emotional state by ELP, according to the study group, after the intervention. There was similarity between the groups in terms of the cut-off point for word frequency and OME. It is noteworthy that the number of categories analysed was higher in the PG compared to the IG.

Table 5: Number of questionnaires, total number of evocations, categories analysed and cut-off points for evocations after the intervention. São Paulo, Brazil, 2022.

	GI	GP
No. of questionnaires	39	35
Questionnaires excluded	0	1
Total number of evocations	195	175
Categories analysed	17	29
Minimum frequency	3 words	2 words
Frequency cut-off point	8	8
OME cut-off point	3	3

When analysing the composition of the Central Core after the intervention (Tables 6 and 7), it was observed that although there was a reduction in the frequency of evocation of the terms most cited before the intervention ("Tired" and "Anxious"), they continued to be present as elements of the Central Core. The term "Worried" moved from the Central Nucleus to the Contrast Zone in the SG. In addition, both groups brought new positive semantic categories. The term "Happy" appeared in the GI and the terms "Calm" and "Hopeful" appeared in the GP. Words in the First Periphery were observed in both groups, which were absent before the intervention.

Central Centre			First Periphery		
Frequency ≥ 8 and OME < 3.0			Frequency ≥ 8 and OME ≥ 3.0		
	Frequency	OME		Frequency	OME
Tired	16	2,3	Confident	13	3,7
Happy	12	2,4	Hopeful	11	3,6
Looking forward to it	10	2,6			
Contrast Zone			Second Periphery		
Frequency < 8 and OME < 3.0			Frequency < 8 and OME ≥ 3.0		
	Frequency	OME		Frequency	OME
Calm down	7	1,9	Relaxed	5	3,2
Worried	7	2,4	Angry	5	3,6
Peaceful	7	2,9	Sleepy	5	3,6
Thank you	5	1,4	Lively	4	4,0
Sad	5	2,0	Pain	3	4,7
In peace	5	2,6			
Anguished	3	2,3			

Chart 7: Composition of the Central Core, Contrast Zone and Peripheries of the GP after the intervention. São Paulo, Brazil, 2022.

Central Centre			First Periphery		
Frequency ≥ 8 and OME < 3.0			Frequency ≥ 8 and OME ≥ 3.0		
	Frequency	OME		Frequency	OME
Tired	16	2,1	Thoughtful	8	3,3
Hopeful	9	2,2			
Peaceful	9	2,3			
Looking forward to it	8	2,9			
Contrast Zone			Second Periphery		
Frequency < 8 and OME < 3.0			Frequency < 8 and OME ≥ 3.0		
	Frequency	OME		Frequency	OME
Calm down	7	2,0	Sad	6	3,3
Happy	7	2,9	Confident	5	3,0
Worried	6	2,0	Faith	4	3,3
In peace	4	2,3	Cheerful	4	3,5
Thank you	3	2,0	Sleepy	4	4,3
Demotivated	3	2,3	Optimistic	3	3,3
Comfortable	2	1,0	Good	2	3,0
Discouraged	2	1,5	Motivated	2	3,0
Tense	2	2,0	Frustrated	2	3,5
			Reflective	2	3,5
			Dissatisfied	2	3,5
			Relaxed	2	4,0
			Lively	2	4,0
			Determined	2	4,5
			Happy	2	4,5

DISCUSSION

Biosociodemographic and professional characteristics

The sociodemographic analysis of the study population showed a predominance of females, over 40 years old and with few children. According to the profile of nursing in Brazil[106-107], despite the growth in male participation in recent years, nursing is still, by tradition and culture, a predominantly female profession, with women making up 85.1 per cent of workers in the area. With regard to marital status, 48.7% of nursing professionals in the country lived with a partner and 38% said they were single[106]. Another study of PHC nursing workers found that 49.6 per cent of those interviewed were married or living with a partner and 44.4 per cent said they were single[108], which differs from the sample in this study in which most of the participants were married or in a stable union. The reason for this difference is probably due to the age group. In this study, most of the participants were over 40 years old, although there is a rejuvenation of nursing, with a total of 61.7% of workers under 40 in the country[106] and 81.2% in PHC[108].

The number of children observed in the study is similar to the 2012 IBGE fertility data for the country (1.8 children), the southeast region and the state of São Paulo (1.7 children)[109], with more recent data from the SEADE Foundation putting the state's fertility rate at 1.6 children[110].

The composition of the team was also in line with the profile of nursing in the country, in which 77% of the professionals belonged to the technical level[106-107]. Some of the professionals at technical level had higher education and specialisation, characterising the overqualification of the workforce, which is the situation in which the individual's educational level, and/or its work experience and/or their skills exceed the needs of the work they do[111]. The overqualification of the workforce is associated with increased access to higher education without an increase in the labour supply for these positions. The percentage of nurses with specialisations in the study is similar to the profile of nursing in the country, which is 80.1% [106].

Regarding time since graduation, the profile of nursing in the country is also showing a process of rejuvenation, with 63.7% of nurses and 49.9% of technical professionals having graduated 10 years or less, which differs from this study in which the majority of professionals had a longer time since graduating. With regard to the length of time they had been working in nursing, the majority of professionals had been working in the area for five years or less, which is different to the national picture, in which only 30 per cent had been working for the same length of time. The discrepancy between time since graduating and time working in nursing can be explained by the difficulty in entering the labour market, especially in the public sector, where the few vacancies are filled and there is no turnover due to the difficulty in setting up new health services and holding competitive examinations[112-113].

Of the study participants, only a small percentage work in the FHS. It's important to note that the two institutions where the research was carried out are mixed basic health units, as they include professionals who work in the ESF and professionals who don't work in this strategy. In Brazil, 2.1% of nursing professionals work in this type of care[106].

With regard to the number of jobs, 63.7% of professionals in the country reported only one job and 25.1% reported two jobs[106], a result similar to that found in this study. Regarding lifestyle habits, the prevalence of participants who declared themselves smokers was similar to the national average of 14.7%. smokers[114], but diverged from the results found for PHC professionals (4.9%)[108]. The results on alcohol consumption were similar to those of a study carried out with primary care nursing workers, in which 82.1% had used alcohol on zero to a maximum of three days in the last month, and 96.2% had used a maximum of two doses in the last month[108]. The low alcohol consumption among the study participants can be explained by the fact that the majority were female, while the prevalence of alcohol abuse in Brazil is higher among males[115].

The health problems under drug treatment most frequently mentioned by the participants were SAH, DM and depression, with prevalences similar to those observed in the country. According to the 2013 National Health Survey, the prevalence of self-reported SAH was 21.4 per cent[116], the prevalence of DM was 9.4 per cent[117] and the prevalence of self-reported depression was 7.6 per cent, with a higher prevalence among women - 10.9 per cent[118].

Most of the participants in the survey reported regular sleep quality, and the average number of hours of sleep per night was lower than that found in a study of PHC nursing professionals, in which 68% of the participants reported sleeping between seven and eight hours every night[108]. Studies on the quality of sleep of nursing workers often focus on professionals who work in hospitals and especially on the night shift, but little is discussed about the sleep of PHC workers. In a study carried out in India, 38.6% of primary care nursing professionals had poor sleep quality[119], and a Brazilian study found that 73% of nurses had poor sleep quality[120].

Characteristics of nursing professionals related to moderating variables

The type of coping most used by the participants was Coping The most used strategies were Planning, followed by Religion and Positive Reinterpretation. The lowest mean scores were found for Coping focused on dysfunctional emotion and the Substance Abuse strategy. A survey of Polish nurses showed similar results, with a higher frequency of problem-focused coping, active coping and planning as the most used strategies and substance abuse as the least used[121]. Another survey of PHC professionals, including nurses, found that the main strategies used were Active Coping, Acceptance and Religion, and the least used was Substance Abuse[122]. A study of nurses working in public health in Jordan found a different result, with the most used strategies being Humour and Emotional support and the least used being Denial[123], which could be attributed to the cultural and religious characteristics of this population. The spiritual well-being of the study participants was classified as moderate. Similar numerical values were observed in a study of Iranian hospital nurses, which showed an average of 94.7 points on the EBE[124]. Slightly lower numerical results were found in a study carried out with Iranian nurses working in university hospitals, whose average scores for the scale and its dimensions were 76.9 on the EBN, 38.3 on the BEE and 38.6 on the BER[125], and with South Korean intensive care nurses, who had an average of 63.2 points on the EBN, 33.8 points on the BEE and 29.3 points on the BER. Even with lower average scores, the results of these studies remain within the classification of moderate spiritual well-being[126]. No studies were found that used the EBE in PHC.

Characteristics of nursing professionals related to outcome variables

With regard to perceived stress, this study showed Similar averages to other studies carried out in Brazil show similar results for stress among primary care nursing workers. In a study carried out with PHC professionals in Sapopemba

(São Paulo), the average perceived stress was 42.2 (±13.9), with the highest scores observed in nurses[127]. Another study of FHS nursing professionals in the municipality of São Paulo (São Paulo) showed an average perceived stress of 44.3 (±13.3) for nurses and 39.0 (±13.7) for nursing assistants[128].

The stress of health professionals, especially nurses, has been highlighted since the advent of the COVID-19 pandemic. Both in Brazil and in other countries, nursing professionals have suffered and are still suffering from high levels of stress, regardless of the segment and level of care in which they work. In a survey carried out in Canada, 82.5% of participants had levels of perceived stress classified as moderate to high[129], with these same levels of stress found in 64.7% of nursing professionals in Colombia[130], 69.7% in Nigeria[131] and 57.3% in Jordan[132]. The average perceived stress in Polish nurses was 20.9 (±5.2) on the PSS-10, with a moderate-high stress classification[133]. Chinese nurses also obtained a moderate-high stress rating on the EEP-10, with an average score above 26 points[134]. Nurses in Iran[135] and Sweden[136] had high levels of perceived stress on the PSS-14, with a mean score of 30.3 (±7.0) and 32.7 respectively. There is no consensus on the results found in clinical trials using flower therapy to reduce stress. A study carried out with teachers found a significant reduction in stress measured with the List of Stress Signs and Symptoms[70], but another study carried out with nursing students did not find significant results in reducing stress measured with the PSS-14[76]. The differences in these results can be explained by the use of individualised formulas in the first study, and the use of a collective formula in the second. Stress at work can lead to the development of negative mood and fatigue[137]. In this study, the dimensions with the highest BRUMS scores were Fatigue and Tension. Studies using the BRUMS to assess mood in nursing professionals are scarce. A clinical trial carried out with nursing professionals working in a cancer hospital in the city of São Paulo (São Paulo, Brazil) found similar results to the present study in the Tension (7.4) and Fatigue (9.6) domains, but with different results for the Vigour (9.9) domain, in which the present study showed lower results[138]. We identified a study with PHC professionals carried out in Spain before the pandemic, in which the POMS was used to assess the emotional state of workers after a mindfulness intervention. In that study, the dimensions with the highest scores were Fatigue-Inertia, with an average of 5.3±2.8 points, and Tension-Anxiety, with an average of 4.7±2.3 points[139]. No studies were found that used Bach flower interventions to improve mood.It is worth pointing out that, according to the analysis of the studies, levels of stress and negative mood in nursing professionals were already high before the pandemic, but have increased even more as a result.

Intervention outcome

In the present study, the flower formula showed no significant difference from the placebo formula in reducing stress levels and improving mood as measured by the EEP-14, BRUMS and ELP instruments. Both GI and GP participants showed positive results at the end of the intervention. The key to the success of an RCT is that the tested intervention has shown efficacy in producing significant values above the placebo effect, especially in PICS[140]. The placebo effect cannot be isolated, because together with the intervention it makes up the total effect of the treatment carried out[141-142]. More than 35 per cent of patients experience therapeutic effects from placebo treatment[141]. The complexity of the placebo effect is due to its multiple components. Social, environmental and contextual factors (culture, therapist-patient relationship, treatment characteristics) shape psychological mechanisms (such as implicit learning, expectation and mental state), which in turn modulate the biological mechanisms that cause the placebo effect(141-).142). This study assessed participants' expectations of the treatment, their perception of the study group to which they were allocated and their perception of change with the use of the bottle they received, in an attempt to identify the influence of the placebo effect on the intervention. Most participants began the study with some expectation of improvement. The highest initial expectations of treatment were reported in the GI, but with no statistically significant difference from the GP. Expectation is part of the psychological mechanisms that make up the placebo effect and is essential for its occurrence. The most important aspect of the expectation of a response to treatment is its tendency to be self-confirming. The strength of the placebo effect is highly correlated with the magnitude of the expectation of response[142]. In the present study, none of the participants reported an expectation of "no improvement" with the use of the bottle they received. Another issue related to expectations is the occurrence of motivational concordance. According to this theory, individuals seek out treatments and therapies that are in line with their beliefs, values and philosophical orientation in life, thus presenting positive expectations regarding the outcome of these practices. For this reason, it can be inferred that people who use PICS tend to are the people who believe in the practices, which leads to a positive expectation of results, inducing the placebo effect[82,143].

At the end of the intervention, most of the participants said they believed they were taking part in the research in the IG, especially those in the IG. One of the reasons that may have influenced participants to this belief was the fact that the label was identified as a "treatment bottle" in both groups, which generated a bias in the study. The relationship between the carer and the recipient of care is therapeutic and can influence the participants' beliefs, expectations and mental state about the process of health and illness. The therapist-patient relationship can affect the incidence of signs and symptoms, both by motivating behavioural changes and by having an impact on psychological mechanisms[141,144]. In this study, contact between the researcher and the participants took place exclusively remotely, using electronic forms and text messages. Even so, at the end of the research, some participants sent messages thanking her for her participation, as they felt "cared for" and "looked after". This feeling of welcome may also have contributed to the development of the placebo effect in the study. Social/observational learning can also interfere with the outcome. One study showed that patients who observed others receiving analgesia experienced a reduction in pain due to the placebo effect[145]. During the intervention, many participants learnt about the research from their colleagues who were already taking part, and who were reporting positive results from using the bottle, which may also have contributed to the manifestation of positive effects even with the use of the placebo formula. The very therapeutic ritual of consuming the placebo can lead individuals to improve their conditions[144].

Although some authors report that the expectation of positive results from an intervention can result in greater adherence to the However, this was not the case in this study, as less than half of the participants used the bottle they received as directed, i.e. four drops, four times a day, five to seven times a week. It could be assumed that the hectic routine of these professionals, consisting of work and household chores, would have interfered with the use of the vials. When analysing the interactions, three variables showed significant results: the BEE domain of the EBE, the coping strategy Acceptance and sleep quality. BEE had a significant influence on all the variables studied. The use of spirituality and religiosity is one of the coping strategies used by nursing professionals to deal with the challenges caused by work overload. Spirituality and religiosity have a positive influence on the physical and mental health of nurses, bringing comfort to stay at work, increasing energy and attention, reducing the emotional burden and deepening the connection with both the patient and co-workers, reducing the perception of stressors in the workplace and contributing to a sense of well-being[147-148].Spirituality, and more specifically BEE, influences mood through the mediating effect of self-esteem and meaning in life. Both self-esteem and meaning of life have a mediating effect between spirituality and positive affect, while self-esteem mediates the effect between spirituality and negative affect[149]. Several studies point to a negative correlation between spiritual well-being and depressive mood[149- 151]. Spirituality helps sustain nurses' sense of purpose, making them more resilient in difficult situations[151], such as the one faced during the COVID-19 pandemic. It is important to emphasise that almost all the participants in the study had moderate to high levels of spiritual well-being. Acceptance coping significantly influenced the levels of perceived stress. Lazarus divided coping strategies into action coping (those that alter the source of stress) and palliative coping (reducing the emotional discomfort caused by the stressor)[152]. Adopting positive coping strategies leads to a reduction in occupational stress, while using negative strategies increases it[122]. It's important to note that healthcare organisations have hierarchies and must follow bureaucratic procedures, which doesn't always allow nurses to use problem-focused coping strategies. For this reason, it is necessary to find ways to deal with the emotional discomfort caused by the situation[152]. Given the lack of control and autonomy brought on by the COVID-19 pandemic, it makes sense that this strategy would significantly influence participants' stress levels. Sleep quality had a significant influence on Depression and Vigour. A good night's sleep has a positive effect on mood[153]. Among the possible causes of sleep disorders in healthcare professionals are high workloads and stress-induced sleep problems. Sleep problems can be associated with depression in a bidirectional relationship[154]. Better mood scores on the BRUMS were found in individuals with good sleep quality. Sleeping well increases vigour and reduces tension and fatigue[153]. There is a negative and significant correlation between pandemic fatigue and sleep quality in nurses[155].

The results found in the ELP analysis were similar to the quantitative results of the analyses of the instruments that assessed the study's outcomes. When looking at the components of the Central Core in the ELP analysis, the terms "Tired" and "Anxious" were the most frequently evoked in both study groups.

Tiredness and fatigue are synonymous and are part of the routine of nursing workers. Evidence suggests that 75 to 80 per cent of nursing professionals in the United States experience high levels of fatigue. of fatigue[156]. Fatigue was already present in nurses' daily lives before the pandemic, but on a smaller scale. In a 2014 survey of nurses working in the ESF in Arapiraca (Alagoas - Brazil), the average score on the Self-Applied Fatigue Questionnaire was 66.8 (±16.6), indicating that signs of fatigue were sometimes or rarely present. This study also showed that the risk of fatigue increased in nurses aged over 32 and with more than seven years of work in nursing, which is the profile of the nurses in the present study[157].

In addition to chronic fatigue, the emergence of the COVID-19 pandemic has also increased anxiety levels among the general population, and especially among health professionals who work directly with infected patients. In POMS, from which BRUMS is derived, the stress domain is directly associated with anxiety[158]. In the BRUMS, the questions in this domain include the manifestations of tension: fear, worry, musculoskeletal tension and anxiety[159]. According to a systematic review and meta-analysis carried out in 2020, the prevalence of anxiety in healthcare professionals was 23.2%[160]. One study showed that of the healthcare professionals who had high levels of fear on the COVID-19 Fear Scale (23.6±6.9), 60% had extremely severe anxiety on the Depression, Anxiety and Stress Scale - DASS-21[161]. In another study, 87.8 per cent of PHC nurses who had altered levels of anxiety on the DASS-21 associated their anxiety with COVID-19[162].

One point that struck me during this research was the number of studies carried out in PHC, which is much lower than those carried out in hospitals and urgent and emergency care centres, as well as interventions focused on reducing stress and improving the mood of professionals working in this sector. PHC has also played an important role during the COVID-19 pandemic, due to its role in educating people about the importance of health. prevention, differential diagnosis of flu-like symptoms, support for vulnerable members of the community and reducing demand on hospitals, as well as maintaining the general health of the population and other issues unrelated to the pandemic, such as chronic diseases and reproductive health[163]. We need to look carefully at this neglect of primary care, given its importance to the country's health system.

Limitations of the study

Despite the care taken in drawing up and applying the protocol for this study, there are some limitations. The use of labelling the vials as "treatment vials" may have contributed to the misconception on the part of the participants that they were taking part in the study in GI, even though they had been advised that neither they nor the researcher would be aware of which study group they would be allocated to. Other factors that may have contributed to the manifestation of the placebo effect in the PG participants include interaction with the therapist, social/observational learning and the characteristics of the treatment, since both the bottle with the flower formula and the bottle with the placebo formula were the same in appearance and taste.

Another important point is the use of a collective formula. Bach florals work best when prescribed according to the individual characteristics and needs of the user, and the use of a collective formula may have reduced the effectiveness of the intervention.

An important issue is the length of time the formula can be used, just four weeks. Although children and more sensitive individuals show faster results with the use of Bach florals[13,59], the literature recommends that adults need at least sixty days of treatment to show results[12]. However, for prolonged use of flower therapy, it is necessary to adjust the formula according to the new needs that have arisen, which would not be possible in this study.

CONCLUSION

According to the results, the flower formula made up of the essences Cherry Plum, Elm, Hornbeam, Olive, Star of Bethlehem, Walnut and White Chestnut showed similar results to the placebo in reducing stress and improving mood. In the intra-group results, both the intervention group and the placebo group showed a significant reduction in levels of perceived stress and an improvement in psycho-emotional states.

REFERENCES

1. Campos JADB, Martins BG, Campos LA, Valadão-Dias FF, Marôco J. Symptoms related to mental disorder in healthcare workers during the COVID-19 pandemic in Brazil. Int Arch Occup Env Health. 2021;94(5):1023-1032. DOI: 10.1007/s00420-021-01656-4

2. Aslan H, Pekince H. Nursing students' views on the COVID-19 pandemic and their percieved stress levels. Perspect Psychiatr Care. 2021;57(2):695-701. DOI: 10.1111/ppc.12597

3. Salari N, Hosseinian-Far A, Jalali R, Vaisi-Raygani A, Rasoupoor S, Mohammadi M, et al. Prevalence of stress, anxiety, depression among the general population during the COVID-19 pandemic: a systematic review and meta-analysis. Global Health. 2020;16(1):57-68. DOI:10.1186/s12992-020-00589-w

4. Torales J, O'Higgins M, Castaldelli-Maia JM, Ventriglio A. The outbreak of COVID-19 coronavirus and its impact on global mental health. Int J Soc Psychiatry. 2020;66(4):317-320. DOI:10.1177/0020764020915212

5. Roberts RK, Grubb PL. The consequences of nursing stress and need for integrated solutions. Rehabil Nurs. 2014;39(2):62-69. DOI:10.1002/rnj.97

6. Al Maqbali M, Al Sinani M, Al-Lenjawi B. Prevalence of stress, depression, anxiety and sleep disturbance among nurses during the COVID-19 pandemic: A systematic review and meta-analysis. J Psychosom Res. 2021;141:110343. DOI: https://doi.org/10.1016/j.jpsychores.2020.110343

7. Kang Y. Psychological stress-induced changes in salivary alpha-amylase and adrenergic activity. Nurs Health Sci. 2010;12(4):477-484. DOI: 10.1111/j.1442-2018.2010.00562.x

8. Yaribeygi H, Panahi Y, Sahraei H, Johnston TP, Sahebkar A. The impact of stress on body function: a review. EXCLI J. 2017;16:1057-1072. DOI: 10.17179/excli2017-480

9. Bekhbat M, Neigh GN. Sex differences in the neuro-immune consequences of stress: Focus on depression and anxiety. Brain Behav Immun. 2018;67:1-12. DOI:10.1016/j.bbi.2017.02.006.

10. Feskanich D, Hastrup JL, Marshall JR, Colditz GA, Stampfer MJ, Willett WC. Stress and suicide in the Nurses' Health Study. J Epidemiol Community Health. 2002;56:95-98. DOI: https://doi.org/10.1136/jech.56.2.95

11. Arruda APCCBN. Effectiveness of Bach florals on the spiritual well-being of university students: Double-blind randomised clinical trial [thesis]. Botucatu: School of Medicine, Universidade Estadual Paulista "Júlio de Mesquita Filho";

2012. Available from: https://repositorio.unesp.br/handle/11449/106069

12. Nascimento VF, Nascimento HF, Silva RGM, Graça BC. Use of Bach florals in holistic psychotherapy. Rev Saúde.com. 2017;13(1):770-778. DOI: 10.22481/rsc.v13i1.367

13. Brazil. Ministry of Health. Ordinance no. 702, of 21 March 2018. Amends Consolidation Ordinance No. 2/GM/MS, of 28 September 2017, to include new practices in the National Policy for Integrative and Complementary Practices. - PNPIC. In: Federal Official Gazette. Brasília; 22 March 2018; Section 1, p.74. Disponível em: https://www.jusbrasil.com.br/diarios/183026231/dou-secao-1-22-03-2018-pg-74

14. Martins JT, Robazzi MLCC, Bobroff MCC. Pleasure and suffering in the work of the nursing team: Reflection in the light of Dejourian psychodynamics. Rev Esc Enferm USP. 2010;44(4):1107-1111. DOI:10.1590/S0080-62342010000400036

15. Duarte JMG, Simões ALA. Meanings of work for nursing professionals at a teaching hospital. Rev enferm UERJ. 2015;23(3):388-394. DOI:10.12957/reuerj.2015.6756

16. Paschoal T, Tamayo A. Validation of the Work Stress Scale. Estud Psicol. 2004;9(1):45-52. DOI:10.1590/s1413-294x2004000100006

17. Hirschle ALT, Gondim SMG. Stress and well-being at work: A literature review. Ciênc saúde coletiva. 2020;25(7):2721-2736. DOI:10.1590/1413-81232020257.27902017

18. Jetha A, Kernan L, Kurowski A. Conceptualising the dynamics of workplace stress: A systems-based study of nursing aides. BMC Health Serv Res. 2017;17(1):1-11. DOI:10.1186/s12913-016-1955-8

19. Teixeira CAB, Pereira SS, Cardoso L, Seleghin MR, Reis LN, Gherardi-Donato ECS. Occupational stress among nursing technicians and assistants: coping focused on the problem. Invest Educ Enferm. 2015;33(1):29-34. DOI: https://doi.org/10.17533/udea.iee.v33n1a04

20. Maharaj S, Lees T, Lal S. Prevalence and risk factors of depression, anxiety, and stress in a cohort of Australian nurses. Int J Environ Res Public Health. 2019;16(1):61. DOI:10.3390/ijerph16010061

21. Biff D, Pires DEP, Forte ECN, Trindade LL, Machado RR, Amadigi FR, et al. Nurses' workload: Lights and shadows in the family health strategy. Ciênc saúde coletiva. 2020;25(1):147-158. DOI:10.1590/1413-81232020251.28622019

22. Almeida LGN, Torres SC, Santos CMF. Occupational risks in the work of primary care health professionals. Rev Enferm Contemp. 2012;1(1):142-

154. DOI:10.17267/2317-3378rec.v1i1.51

23. Silva RM, Goulart CT, Guido LA. Historical evolution of the concept of stress. Rev Cient Sena Aires. 2018;7(2):148-156. Available at: http://revistafacesa.senaaires.com.br/index.php/revisa/article/viewFile/316/225

24. Sousa MBC, Silva HPA, Galvão-Coelho NL. Response to stress: I. Homeostasis and allostasis theory. Estud psicol. 2015;20(1):2-11. DOI: 10.5935/1678-4669.20150002

25. Freitas PM, Rocha CM, Silva TCC. A theoretical study on the Cognitive Model of Stress and Coping. Revise. 2010;1:1-19. DOI: https://doi.org/10.46635/revise.v1i01-01.1650

26. Lazarus RS, Folkman S. Stress, appraisal, and coping. New York: Springer; 1984. 460 p.

27. Folkman S, Lazarus RS, Gruen RJ, DeLongis A. Appraisal, coping, health status, and psychological symptoms. J Pers Soc Psychol. 1986;50(3):571-579. DOI:10.1037/0022-3514.50.3.571

28. Folkman S, Lazarus RS, Dunkel-Schetter C, DeLongis A, Gruen RJ. Dynamics of a stressful encounter: Cognitive appraisal, coping, and cncounter outcomes. J Pers Soc Psychol. 1986;50(5):992-1003. DOI: https://doi.org/10.1037//0022- 3514.50.5.992

29. Dias EN, Pais-Ribeiro JL. The Folkman and Lazarus coping model: historical and conceptual aspects. Rev Psicol Saúde. 2019;11(2):55-66. DOI: 10.20435/pssa.v11i2.642

30. Folkman S. Stress, coping, and hope. Psychooncology. 2010;19:901-908. DOI:10.1002/pon.1836

31. Baldacchino D, Draper P. Spiritual coping strategies: A review of the nursing research literature. J Adv Nurs. 2001;34(6):833-841. DOI:10.1046/j.1365- 2648.2001.01814.x

32. Pedrão RB, Beresin R. Nursing and spirituality. Einstein (São Paulo). 2010;8(1 Pt 1):86-91. DOI:10.1590/s1679-45082010ao1208

33. Guimarães HP, Avezum A. The impact of spirituality on physical health. Rev Psiquiatr Clin. 2007;34(SUPPL. 1):88-94. DOI:10.1590/S0101-60832007000700012

34. Saad M, Masiero D, Battistella LR. Evidence-based spirituality. Acta Fisiátrica. 2001;8(3):18-23. DOI:10.5935/0104-7795.20010003

35. Forti S, Serbena CA, Scaduto AA. Spirituality/religiousity measurement and health in Brazil: A systematic review. Ciênc saúde coletiva. 2020;25(4):1463-1474. DOI:10.1590/1413-81232020254.21672018

36. Lucchetti G, Koenig HG, Lucchetti ALG. Spirituality, religiousness, and

mental health: A review of the current scientific evidence. World J Clin Cases. 2021;9(26):7620-7631. DOI:10.12998/wjcc.v9.i26.7620

37. Alharbi H, Alshehry A. Perceived stress and coping strategies among ICU nurses in government tertiary hospitals in Saudi Arabia: A cross-sectional study. Ann Saudi Med. 2019;39(1):48-55. DOI:10.5144/0256-4947.2019.48

38. Tuck I, Alleyne R, Thinganjana W. Spirituality and stress management in healthy adults. J Holist Nurs. 2006;24(4):245-253. DOI: 10.1177/0898010106289842

39. De-Souza MM, Garbeloto M, Denez K, Eger-Mangrich I. Evaluation of the central effects of Bach florals in mice using specific pharmacological models. Rev Bras Farmacogn. 2006;16(3):365-371. DOI: 10.1590/s0102-695x2006000300014

40. Arruda APN, Balneaves LG, Turrini RNT. Bach flowers in a patient with a history of sexual abuse: a case report. Cad Naturol Ter Complem. 2015;4(6):67-75. DOI: https://doi.org/10.19177/cntc.v4e6201567-75

41. Resende MMC, Costa FEC, Gardona RGB, Araújo RG, Mundim FGL, Costa MJC. Preventive use of bach flower rescue remedy in the control of risk factors for cardiovascular disease in rats. Complement Ther Med. 2014;22(4):719-723. DOI:10.1016/j.ctim.2014.06.008

42. Asher GN, Gerkin J, Gaynes BN. Complementary therapies for mental health disorders. Med Clin North Am. 2017;101(5):847-864. DOI: 10.1016/j.mcna.2017.04.004

43. Jesus E, Nascimento M. Bach Flowers: a natural medicine in practice. Rev Enferm UNISA. 2005;6(1):32-37. Available at https://www.ufjf.br/proplamed/files/2013/01/2005-05.pdf

44. Monari C. Participating in life with Bach's florals: A mythological and practical vision. 6th ed. São Paulo: Acallanto; 2018. 782 p.

45. Barnard J. A guide to Dr Bach's flower remedies. 12th ed. São Paulo: Editora Pensamento; 1997. 74 p.

46. Gimenes OMP, Silva MJP, Benko MA. Flower essences: a vibrational intervention with diagnostic and therapeutic possibilities. Rev Esc Enferm USP. 2004;38(4):386-395. DOI:10.1590/s0080-62342004000400004

47. Bach E. Dr Bach's flower remedies. 19th ed. São Paulo: Pensamento; 2006. 96 p.

48. Scheffer M. Dr Bach's flower therapy - Theory and practice. 1st ed. São Paulo: Editora Pensamento; 1991. 229 p.

49. Halberstein RA, Sirkin A, Ojeda-Vaz MM. When less is better: A comparison of Bach® Flower Remedies and Homeopathy. Ann Epidemiol.

2010;20(4):298-307. DOI:10.1016/j.annepidem.2009.11.006

50. Rajendran ES. An evaluation of Avogadro's number in the light of HRTEM and EDS studies of high dilutions of Ferrum metallicum 6, 30, 200, 1M, 10M and 50Mc. Int J High Dilution Res. 2015;14(3):3-9. DOI: https://doi.org/10.51910/ijhdr.v14i3.764

51. Upadhyay RP, Nayak C. Homeopathy emerging as nanomedicine. Int J High DilutionRes. 2011;10(37):299-310. DOI: https://doi.org/10.1016%2Fj.eujim.2012.11.002

52. Fusco SDFB, Pancieri AP, Amancio SCP, Fusco DR, Padovani CR, Minicucci MF, et al. Efficacy of flower therapy for anxiety in overweight or obese adults: A randomised placebo-controlled clinical trial. J Altern Complement Med. 2021;27(5):416-422. DOI:10.1089/acm.2020.0305

53. Ullman D. Exploring possible mechanisms of hormesis and homeopathy in the light of nanopharmacology and ultra-high dilutions. Dose-Response. 2021;19(2):1-13. DOI:10.1177/15593258211022983

54. Bell IR, Ives JA, Jonas WB. Nonlinear effects of nanoparticles: Biological variability from hormetic doses, small particle sizes, and dynamic adaptive interactions. Dose-Response. 2014;12(2):202-232. DOI:10.2203/dose-response.13-025.Bell

55. Bell IR, Koithan M. A model for homeopathic remedy effects: Low dose nanoparticles, allostatic cross-adaptation, and time-dependent sensitisation in a complex adaptive system. BMC Complement Altern Med. 2012;12:191. DOI:10.1186/1472-6882-12-191

56. Howard J. Do Bach flower remedies have a role to play in pain control?. A critical analysis investigating therapeutic value beyond the placebo effect, and the potential of Bach flower remedies as a psychological method of pain relief. Complement Ther Clin Pract. 2007;13(3):174-183. DOI:10.1016/j.ctcp.2007.03.001

57. Rivas-Suárez SR, Águila-Vázquez JA, Suárez-Rodríguez B, Vásquez-Leo L, Casanova-Giral M, Morales-Morales R, et al. Exploring the effectiveness of external use of Bach Flower Remedies on carpal tunnel syndrome: A pilot study. J Evidence-Based Complementary Altern Med. 2017;22(1):18-24. DOI:10.1177/2156587215610705

58. Libster MM. Gentle remedies: Restoring faith in the first step of nonpharmacological infant mental health care for the prevention and treatment of "disruptive behaviour." Arch Psychiatr Nurs. 2019;33(3):299-306. DOI: 10.1016/j.apnu.2019.02.004

59. Gava FGS, Turrini RNT. The use of Bach Flowers to manage the symptoms

of childhood autism: Experience report. Rev Paul Enferm. 2019;30. DOI:10.33159/25959484.repen.2019v30a6

60. Milanés MG, Carpio MHC, RamosMRM, Magluen CM, Varona B. Clinical behaviour of childhood fear of stomatology with Bach flower treatment. Ver Cubana Estomatol. 2018;44(3). Available at: http://scielo.sld.cu/scielo.php?script=sci_arttext&pid=S0034-75072007000300010&lng=es

61. Halberstein R, Desantis L, Sirkin A, Padron-Fajardo V, Ojeda-Vaz M. Healing with Bach ® Flower Essences: Testing a complementary therapy. Complement Health PractRev.2007;12(1):3-14.

62. Salles LF, Silva MJP. Effect of flower essences in anxious individuals. ACTA Paul Enferm. 2012;25(2):238-242. DOI:10.1590/s0103-21002012000200013

63. Docal BP, Mengana LMJ, García EN, Contreras AJD. Andropause and flower therapy. RevCuba Plants Medicinales. 2007;12(3). Available at: http://scielo.sld.cu/scielo.php?script=sci_arttext&pid=S1028-47962007000300003&lng=es&nrm=iso&tlng=es

64. Masi MP. Bach flower therapy in the treatment of chronic major depressive disorder. Altern Ther Health Med. 2003;9(6):108-110. PMID: 14618865

65. Walton SM, Pérez CAS. Bach flower therapy and psychological counselling in women victims of psychological violence. Rev Ciencias Médicas. 2019;23(6):792-798. Available at: http://scielo.sld.cu/scielo.php?script=sci_arttext&pid=S1561-31942019000600792

66. Contrera Vega N, Cedeño Rodríguez E, Vázquez Sánchez M. Efectividad de la terapia floral de Bach en pacientes con alcoholismo crónico. Medisan. 2012;16(4):519-525. Available at: http://scielo.sld.cu/scielo.php?script=sci_arttext&pid=S1029-30192012000400005

67. Lara SRG, Magaton APS, Cesar MBN, Gabrielloni MC, Barbieri M. Experience of women in labour with the use of flower essences. Rev Fun Care Online. 2020;12:162-168. DOI:10.9789/2175-5361.rpcfo.v12.7178

68. Rodríguez-Martín BC. Bach Flower Essences: Effect of White Chestnut on unwanted intrusive thoughts. Rev Cubana Invest Bioméd 2012; 31(2). Available at: http://scielo.sld.cu243

69. Yang SW, Koo M, Wang Y-H. The influence of Bach Rescue Remedy on the autonomic response to mental hallenge in healthy Taiwanese women. Integr Med Res. 2015;4(1):84. DOI:10.1016/j.imr.2015.04.127

70. Pinto RH, Sousa SM, Santos CR, Senna SM, Leal LP, Vasconcelos EMR. Effect of flower therapy on teacher stress: Randomised clinical trial. Rev Min Enferm. 2020;24:e-1318. DOI:10.5935/1415-2762.20200055

71. Suárez SR, Díaz A, Machado FB. Preclinical effect of the Bach flower essence in acute inflammation. Rev Cuba Investig Biomédicas. 2013;32(1):65-73. Available at: https://www.medigraphic.com/pdfs/revcubinvbio/cib-2013/cib131g.pdf

72. Morais AJC, Cerutti ML, Dullius C, Arruda G, Cordova CMM, Valente C. Floral Rescue: An analysis of the effects of flower essence on biochemical components of healthy rats. Cad Naturol Ter Complem. 2022;11(20). Available at: https://portaldeperiodicos.animaeducacao.com.br/index.php/CNTC/article/view/12200

73. Muhlack S, Lemmer W, Klotz P, Müller T, Klieser E. Anxiolytic effect of Rescue Remedy for psychiatric patients. J Clin Psychopharmacol. 2006;26(5):541-542. DOI: 10.1097/01.jcp.0000231608.83520.a1

74. Armstrong NC, Ernst E. A randomised, double-blind, placebo-controlled trial of a Bach Flower Remedy. Complement Ther Nurs Midwifery. 2001;7(4):215-221. DOI:10.1054/ctnm.2001.0525

75. Walach H, Rilling C, Engelke U. Efficacy of Bach-flower remedies in test anxiety: A double-blind, placebo-controlled, randomised trial with partial crossover. J Anxiety Disord. 2001;15(4):359-366. DOI:10.1016/S0887-6185(01)00069-X

76. Albuquerque LMNF, Turrini RNT. Effects of flower essences on nursing students' stress symptoms: a randomised clinical trial. Rev Esc Enferm USP. 2021;56:e20210307. DOI:10.1590/1980-220X-REEUSP-2021-0307

77. Ernst E. Bach flower remedies: A systematic review of randomised clinical trials. Swiss Med Wkly. 2010;140:w13079. DOI:10.4414/smw.2010.13079

78. Thaler K, Kaminski A, Chapman A, Langley T, Gartlehner G. Bach flower remedies for psychological problems and pain: A systematic review. BMC Complement Altern Med. 2009;9:16. DOI:10.1186/1472-6882-9-16

79. Bhide A, Shah PS, Acharya G. A simplified guide to randomised controlled trials. Acta Obstet Gynecol Scand. 2018;97(4):380-387. DOI:10.1111/AOGS.13309

80. Ka Shing L, Loudon K, Treweek S, Sullivan F, Donnan P, Thorpe KE, et al. The PRECIS-2 tool: designing trials that are fit for purpose. BMJ. 2015;350(h2147):1-5. DOI:10.1136/bmj.h2147

81. Williams HC, Burden-Teh E, Nunn AJ. What is a pragmatic clinical trial? J

Invest Dermatol. 2015;135:e33. DOI:10.1038/jid.2015.134

82. Hyland ME, Whalley B. Motivational concordance: An important mechanism in self-help therapeutic rituals involving inert (placebo) substances. J Psychosom Res. 2008;65(5):405-413. DOI:10.1016/j.jpsychores.2008.02.006

83. Salari N, Khazaie H, Hosseinian-Far A, Khaledi-Paveh B, Kazeminia M, Mohammadi M, et al. The prevalence of stress, anxiety and depression within front-line healthcare workers caring for COVID-19 patients: a systematic review and meta-regression. Hum Resour Health. 2020;18(1):1-14. DOI:10.1186/s12960-020-00544-1

84. Mantle F. Bach flower remedies. Complement Ther Nurs Midwifery. 1997;3(5):142-144. DOI:10.1016/S1353-6117(97)80015-7

85. Nosow SKC, Ceolim MF. Selection of Bach florals to improve sleep quality. Rev enferm UFPE on line. 2016;10(Suppl. 4):3662-3668. DOI:10.5205/reuol.9681-89824-1-ED.1004sup201618

86. Luft CDB, Sanches SO, Mazo GZ, Andrade A. Brazilian version of the Perceived Stress Scale: Translation and validation for the elderly. Rev Saude Publica. 2007;41(4):606-615. DOI:10.1590/s0034-89102007000400015

87. Bardaquim VA, Santos SVM, Dias EG, Dalri RCMB, Mendes AMOC, Gallani MC, et al. Stress and cortisol levels among members of the nursing team. Rev Bras Enferm. 2020;73 1(Suppl 1):e20180953. DOI:10.1590/0034-7167-2018- 0953

88. Faro A. Confirmatory factor analysis of the three versions of the Perceived Stress Scale (PSS): A population-based study. Psychol Reflex Crit. 2015;28(1):21-30. DOI:10.1590/1678-7153.201528103

89. Oliveira FJS, Almeida LY, Oliveira JL, Almeida LC, Souza J. Work and mood among public university employees. Rev enferm UERJ. 2019;27:E41794. DOI:10.12957/reuerj.2019.41794

90. Rohlfs ICPM, Rotta TM, Luft CB, Andrade A, Krebs RJ, Carvalho T. The Brunel Mood Scale (Brums): An instrument for early detection of overtraining syndrome. Rev Bras Med Esporte. 2008;14(3):176-181. DOI:10.1590/S1517-86922008000300003

91. Rohlfs ICPM. Validation of the BRUMS test for mood assessment in Brazilian athletes and non-athletes [dissertation]. Florianópolis: Centre f o r Physical Education and Sports, Santa Catarina State University; 2006. Available at: https://sistemabu.udesc.br/pergamumweb/vinculos/00006b/00006bbe.pdf

92. Coutinho M. The free word association technique through the prism of the Tri-Deux-Mots software (version 5.2). Rev Campo do Saber. 2017;3(1):219-243. Available at:

https://periodicos.iesp.edu.br/index.php/campodosaber/article/view/72

93. Silva FD, Apostolidis T, Ferreira MA. Social representations of nursing students on the rights of health users. Rev Bras Enferm. 2020;73(6):e20190510. DOI:10.1590/0034-7167-2019-0510

94. Maroco J, Campos JB, Bonafé FS, Vinagre MG, Pais-Ribeiro J. Brazil-Portugal cross-cultural adaptation of the Brief Cope scale for higher education students. Psicol Saúde e Doenças. 2014;15(2):300-313. DOI: http://dx.doi.org/10.15309/14psd150201

95. Brasileiro SV. Cross-cultural adaptation and psychometric properties of the COPE Breve in a Brazilian sample [dissertation]. Goiânia: Federal University of Goiás; 2012. Available at: https://repositorio.bc.ufg.br/tede/bitstream/tede/3351/5/Dissertação - Sarah Vieira Brasileiro - 2012.pdf

96. Marques LF, Sarriera JC, Dell'Aglio DD. Adaptation and validation of the Spiritual Well-being Scale Well-being Scale(EBE). Psychological Psicológica. 2009;8(2):179-186. Available at: http://pepsic.bvsalud.org/scielo.php?script=sci_arttext&pid=S1677-04712009000200004

97. Gueorguieva R, Krystal JH. Move over ANOVA: Progress in analysing repeated measures data and its reflection in papers published in the Archives of General Psychiatry. Arch Gen Psychiatry. 2004;61(3):310-317. DOI: 10.1001/ARCHPSYC.61.3.310

98. Espírito-Santo H, Daniel F. Calculating and reporting effect sizes on scientific papers (3): Guide to report regression models and ANOVA effect sizes. Rev Port Investig Comport e Soc. 2018;4(1):43-60. DOI: 10.7342/ismt.rpics.2018.4.1.72

99. Wachelke J, Wolter R. Criteria for constructing and reporting prototypical analysis for social representations. Psic: Teor e Pesq. 2011;27(4):521-526. DOI: 10.1590/S0102-37722011000400017

100. Souza TC. Social representations of science: a study from a degree course in biological sciences [dissertation]. São Carlos: Centre for Education and Human Sciences; 2020. Available at: https://repositorio.ufscar.br/bitstream/handle/ufscar/12475/SOUZA_Tamires_2020.pdf?sequence=1&isAllowed=y

101. Sant'Anna HC. openEvoc: A programme to support research into Social Representations. In: Avelar L, Ciscon-Evangelista M, Nardi M, Nascimento A, Neto P, organisers. Social Psychology: Contemporary Challenges. Vitória: GM Gráfica e Editora; 2012. p. 94-103.

102. Faria ACO, Almeida MN. Free recall of words as a diagnostic assessment tool. Rev Educ Pública. 2020;20(38):1-8. DOI: 10.18264/REP

103. Ferreira VCP, Santos Jr. AF, Azevedo RC, Valverde G. The social representation of work: a contribution to the study of motivation. Estação científica. 2005;1:1-13. Available at: https://portal.estacio.br/media/4394/6-a-representacao-social-trabalho- contribuicao-estudo-motivacao.pdf

104. Wolter RMCP, Peixoto ARS, Oliveira FC, Santin TR. Free evocations and prototypical analysis for social thought studies. In: Soares AB, Medeiros CAC, Jardim MEM, Silva MLR, Alves PRSS, Ribeiro R, organisers. Qualitative methodology: Research techniques and examples. 1st ed. Curitiba: Appris; 2022. p. 243-262.

105. Oliveira DC, Marques SC, Gomes AMT, Teixeira MCTV. Analysis of free evocations: A technique for structural analysis of Social Representations. In: Moreira ASPM, Camargo BV, Jesuíno JC, Nóbrega SM, organisers. Theoretical and Methodological Perspectives on Social Representations. João Pessoa: Editora Universitária UFPB; 2005. p. 573-603.

106. Machado MH (Coord). Profile of Nursing in Brazil: Final Report. Rio de Janeiro; 2017. Available from: http://www.cofen.gov.br/perfilenfermagem/pdfs/relatoriofinal.pdf

107. Machado MH, Aguiar Filho W, Lacerda WF, Oliveira E, Lemos W, Wermelinger M, et al. General characteristics of nursing: the socio-demographic profile. Enferm Foco. 2015;6(4):11-17. Available at: http://revista.cofen.gov.br/index.php/enfermagem/article/view/686/296

108. Hidalgo KD, Mielke GI, Parra DC, Lobelo F, Simões EJ, Gomes GO, et al. Health promoting practices and personal lifestyle behaviours of Brazilian health professionals. BMC Public Health. 2016;16(1):1114. DOI: 10.1186/s12889-016- 3778-2

109. Brazilian Institute of Geography and Statistics. Demographic Indicators: Total Fertility Rate. Brazil; 2012. Available from: http://tabnet.datasus.gov.br/cgi/idb2012/a05b.htm

110. State Data Analysis System Foundation. Between 2000 and 2020, the average number of children went from 2.08 children per woman to 1.56. Available at: https://www.seade.gov.br/entre-2000-e-2020-o-numero-medio-de-filhos- went-from-208-children-per-woman-to-156/

111. Chen G, Tang Y, Su Y. The effect of perceived over-qualification on turnover intention from a cognition perspective. Front Psychol. 2021;12. DOI: 10.3389/fpsyg.2021.699715

112. Oliveira JSA, Pires DEP, Alvarez AM, Sena RR, Medeiros SM, Andrade

SR. Trends in the labour market for nurses in the view of managers. Rev Bras Enferm. 2018;71(1):148-155. Available at: https://www.scielo.br/j/reben/a/g3MpJvgbPDsmkfndDH9hjpR/?lang=pt&format = pdf

113. Silva DA, Marcolan JF. Unemployment and psychological distress in nurses. Rev Bras Enferm. 2015;68(5):493-500. DOI:10.1590/0034-7167.20156805502i

114. Malta DC, Vieira ML, Szwarcwald CL, Caixeta R, Brito SMF, Reis AAC. Smoking trends in the Brazilian population according to the 2008 National Household Sample Survey and the 2013 National Health Survey. Rev Bras Epidemiol. 2015;18:45-56. DOI:10.1590/1980-5497201500060005

115. Silva LES, Helman B, Silva DCL, Aquino EC, Freitas PC, Santos RO, et al. Prevalence of heavy episodic drinking in the Brazilian adult population: National Health Survey 2013 and2019. Epidemiole Serv Saude. 2022;31(Special Issue 1):1-15. DOI:10.1590/SS2237-9622202200003.especial

116. Malta DC, Gonçalves RPF, Machado IE, Freitas MIF, Azeredo C, Szwarcwald CL. Prevalence of hypertension according to different diagnostic criteria. National Health Survey. Rev Bras Epidemiol. 2018;21. DOI:10.1590/1980-549720180021.supl.1

117. Muzy J, Campos MR, Emmerick I, Silva RS, Schramm JMA. Prevalence of diabetes mellitus and its complications and characterisation of healthcare gaps based on triangulation of studies. Cad Saude Publica. 2021;37(5). DOI: 10.1590/0102-311X00076120

118. Stopa SR, Malta DC, Oliveira MM, Lopes CS, Menezes PR, Kinoshita RT. Prevalence of self-reported depression in Brazil: Results from the National Health Survey, 2013. Rev Bras Epidemiol. 2015;18:170-180. DOI: 10.1590/1980-5497201500060015

119. Yella T, D'mello MK. Burnout and sleep quality among community health workers during the pandemic in selected city of Andhra Pradesh. Clin Epidemiol Glob Health. 2022;16:101 109. DOI: 10.1016/J.CEGH.2022.101109

120. Silveira FBCA, Lira Neto JCG, Weiss C, Araújo MFM. Association between community and workplace violence and sleep quality among health professionals: A cross-sectional study. Ciênc Saúde Colet. 2021;26(5):1647-1656. DOI:10.1590/1413-81232021265.04522021

121. Stefanowicz-Bielska A, Słomion M, Rąpała M. Analysis of strategies for managing stress by Polish nurses during the COVID-19 pandemic. Healthcare. 2022;10(10):2008. DOI:10.3390/healthcare10102008

122. Aryal S, D'mello MK. Occupational stress and coping strategy among

community health workers of Mangalore Taluk, Karnataka. Indian J Public Health. 2020;64(4):351-356. DOI:10.4103/ijph.IJPH_549_19

123. Alkhawaldeh JM, Soh KL, Mukhtar F, Peng OC, Alkhawaldeh HM, Al-Amer R, et al. Stress management training programme for stress reduction and coping improvement in public health nurses: A randomized controlled trial. J Adv Nurs. 2020;76(11):3123-3135. DOI:10.1111/jan.14506

124. Soleimani MA, Sharif SP, Yaghoobzadeh A, Sheikhi MR, Panarello B, Win MTM. Spiritual well-being and moral distress among Iranian nurses. Nurs Ethics. 2019;26(4):1101-1113. DOI:10.1177/0969733016650993

125. Jafari M, Fallahi-Khoshknab M. Competence in providing spiritual care and its relationship with spiritual well-being among Iranian nurses. J Educ Health Promot. 2021;10:388. DOI:10.4103/jehp.jehp

126. Kim HS, Yeom HA. The association between spiritual well-being and burnout in intensive care unit nurses: A descriptive study. Intensive Crit Care Nurs. 2018;46:92-97. DOI:10.1016/j.iccn.2017.11.005

127. Atanes ACM, Andreoni S, Hirayama MS, Montero-Marin J, Barros VV, Ronzani TM, et al. Mindfulness, perceived stress, and subjective well-being: A correlational study in primary care health professionals. BMC Complement Altern Med. 2015;15:303. DOI:10.1186/s12906-015-0823-0

128. Leonelli LB, Andreoni S, Martins P, Kozasa EH, De Salvo VL, Sopezki D, et al. Perceived stress in family health strategy professionals. Rev Bras Epidemiol. 2017;20(2):286-298. DOI:10.1590/1980-5497201700020009

129. El Gindi H, Shalaby R, Gusnowski A, Vuong W, Surood S, Hrabok M, et al. The mental health impact of the COVID-19 pandemic among physicians, nurses, and other health care providers in Alberta: Cross-sectional survey. JMIR Form Res. 2022;6(3):e27469. DOI:10.2196/27469

130. Guillen-Burgos HF, Gomez-Ureche J, Renowitzky C, Acevedo-Vergara K, Perez-Florez M, Villalba E, et al. Prevalence and associated factors of mental health outcomes among healthcare workers in Northern Colombia: A cross-sectional and multi-centre study. J Affect Disord Reports. 2022;10:100415. DOI:10.1016/j.jadr.2022.100415

131. Olude OA, Odeyemi K, Kanma-Okafor OJ, Badru OA, Bashir SA, Olusegun JO, et al. Mental health status of doctors and nurses in a Nigerian tertiary hospital: A COVID-19 experience. S Afr J Psychiat. 2022;28:1904. DOI:10.4102/sajpsychiatry.v28i0.1904

132. Al Hadid LAE, Al Barmawi MA, Alnjadat R, Farajat LAl. The impact of stress associated with caring for patients with COVID-19 on career decisions, resilience, and perceived self-efficacy in newly hired nurses in Jordan: A cross-sectional study. Health Sci Rep. 2022;5(6):e899. DOI:10.1002/hsr2.899

133.	Sierakowska M, Doroszkiewicz H. Stress coping strategies used by nurses during the COVID-19 pandemic. PeerJ. 2022;10:e13288.DOI:10.7717/peerj.13288

134.	Zhou Y, Wang Y, Huang M, Wang C, Pan Y, Ye J, et al. Psychological stress and psychological support of chinese nurses during severe public health events. BMC Psychiatry. 2022;22:800. DOI:10.1186/s12888-022-04451-8

135.	Amjadi S, Mohammadi S, Khojastehrad A. Perceived stress and quality of life among frontline nurses fighting against COVID-19: A web-based cross-sectional study. J Educ Health Promot. 2022;11:128. DOI: 10.4103/jehp.jehp_175_21

136.	Skogevall S, Holmström IK, Kaminsky E, Håkansson Eklund J. Telephone nurses' perceived stress, self-efficacy and empathy in their work with frequent callers. Nurs Open. 2022;9(2):1394-1401. DOI:10.1002/nop2.889

137.	Martínez-Zaragoza F, Fernández-Castro J, Benavides-Gil G, García-Sierra R. How the lagged and accumulated effects of stress, coping, and tasks affect mood and fatigue during nurses' shifts. Int J Env Res Public Health. 2020;17(19):7277. DOI:10.3390/ijerph17197277

138.	Silva NO, Kuba G, Kurebayashi LFS, Turrini RNT. Effect of Chinese auriculotherapy on the mood of health professionals: a pilot study. Rev Enferm UFSM. 2021;11(e53). DOI:10.5902/21797692618883

139.	Asuero AM, Blanco TR, Pujol-Ribera E, Berenguera A, Queraltó JM. Evaluation of the effectiveness of a mindfulness programme in primary care professionals. Gac Sanit. 2013;27(6):521-528. DOI: https://doi.org/10.1016%2Fj.aprim.2017.03.009

140.	Kong J, Kaptchuk TJ, Polich G, Kirsch I, Vangel M, Zyloney C, et al. Expectancy and treatment interactions: A dissociation between acupuncture analgesia and expectancy evoked placebo analgesia. Neuroimage. 2009;45(3):940-949. DOI:10.1016/j.neuroimage.2008.12.025141.

141.	Zion SR, Crum AJ. Mindsets matter: A new framework for harnessing the placebo effect in modern medicine. Int Rev Neurobiol. 2018;138:137-160. DOI:10.1016/bs.irn.2018.02.002

142.	Kirsch I. Response expectancy and the placebo effect. Int Rev Neurobiol. 2018;138:81-93. DOI:10.1016/bs.irn.2018.01.003

143.	Rodríguez-Martín BC, Fallas-Durán M, Gaitskell B, Vega-Rojas D, Martínez- Chaigneau P. Predictors of positive opinion about Bach Flower Remedies in adults from three Latin-American countries: An exploratory study. Complement Ther Clin Pract. 2017;27:52-56. DOI:10.1016/j.ctcp.2017.04.002

144.	Kaptchuk TJ, Kelley JM, Conboy LA, Davis RB, Kerr CE, Jacobson EE, et al. Components of placebo effect: Randomised controlled trial in patients with irritable bowel syndrome. BMJ. 2008;336(7651):999-1003. DOI:10.1136/be

145. Colloca L, Benedetti F. Placebo analgesia induced by social observational learning. Pain. 2009;144:28-34. DOI:10.1016/j.pain.2009.01.033

146. Hoffmann TC, Del Mar C. Patients' expectations of the benefits and harms of treatments, screening, and tests: A systematic review. JAMA Intern Med. 2015;175(2):274-286. DOI:10.1001/jamainternmed.2014.6016

147. Diego-Cordero R, Iglesias-Romo M, Badanta B, Lucchetti G, Vega-Escaño J. Burnout and spirituality among nurses: A scoping review. Explore. 2022;18(5):612-620. DOI:10.1016/j.explore.2021.08.001

148. Campbell D. Spirituality, stress, and retention of nurses in critical care. Dimens Crit Care Nurs. 2013;32(2):78-83. DOI: 10.1097/DCC.0b013e31828083a4

149. Craig DJ, Fardouly J, Rapee RM. The effect of spirituality on mood: Mediation by self-esteem, social support, and meaning in life. J Relig Health. 2022;61(1):228-251. DOI:10.1007/s10943-021-01342-2

150. Ata G, Kılıç D. Correlation of spiritual well-being with hope and depression in oncology patients: The case of Turkey. Perspect Psychiatr Care. 2022;58(4):1460-1466. DOI:10.1111/ppc.12950

151. Batalla VRD, Barrameda ALN, Basal JMS, Bathan ASJ, Bautista JEG, Rebueno MCDR, et al. Moderating effect of occupational stress on spirituality and depression of Registered Nurses in tertiary hospital: A structural equation model. J Adv Nurs. 2019;75(4):772-782. DOI: 10.1111/jan.13856

152. Dewe PJ. Stressor frequency, tension, tiredness and coping: some measurement issues and a comparison across nursing groups. J Adv Nurs. 1989;14(4):308-320. DOI:10.1111/j.1365-2648.1989.tb03418.x

153. Ferreira TS, Moreira CZ, Guo J, Noce F. Effects of a 12-hour shift on mood states and sleepiness of neonatal intensive care unit nurses. Rev Esc Enferm USP. 2017;51:e03202. DOI:10.1590/S1980-220X2016033203202

154. Marvaldi M, Mallet J, Dubertret C, Moro MR, Guessoum SB. Anxiety, depression, trauma-related, and sleep disorders among healthcare workers during the COVID-19 pandemic: A systematic review and meta-analysis.Neurosci Biobehav Rev. 2021;126:252-264. DOI:10.1016/j.neubiorev.2021.03.024

155. Labrague LJ. Pandemic fatigue and clinical nurses' mental health, sleep quality and job contentment during the covid-19 pandemic: The mediating role of resilience. J Nurs Manag. 2021;29(7):1992-2001. DOI: 10.1111/jonm.13383

156. Cochran KR. An examination of work characteristics, fatigue, and recovery among acute care nurses. JONA. 2021;51(2):89-94. DOI: 10.1097/NNA.0000000000000975

157. Almeida LMWS. Fatigue at work in Family Health Strategy nurses [thesis]. Ribeirão Preto: University of São Paulo School of Nursing; 2014. Available at: https://teses.usp.br/teses/disponiveis/83/83131/tde-20022015-161019/publico/LENIRAMARIAWANDERLEYSANTOSDEALMEIDA.pdf

158. Samaha E, Lal S, Samaha N, Wyndham J. Psychological, lifestyle and coping contributors to chronic fatigue in shift-worker nurses. J Adv Nurs. 2007;59(3):221-232. DOI:10.1111/j.1365-2648.2007.04338.x

159. Brandt R, Herrero D, Massetti T, Crocetta TB, Guarnieri R, Monteiro CBM, et al. The Brunel mood scale rating in mental health for physically active and apparently healthy populations. Health. 2016;8(2):125-132. DOI: 10.4236/health.2016.82015

160. Pappa S, Ntella V, Giannakas T, Giannakoulis VG, Papoutsi E, Katsaounou P. Prevalence of depression, anxiety, and insomnia among healthcare workers during the COVID-19 pandemic: A systematic review and meta-analysis. Brain Behav Immun. 2020;88:901-907. DOI:10.1016/j.bbi.2020.05.026

161. Alnazly E, Khraisat OM, Al-Bashaireh AM, Bryant CL. Anxiety, depression, stress, fear and social support during COVID-19 pandemic among Jordanian healthcare workers.PLoS One. 2021;16(3):e0247679. DOI: 10.1371/journal.pone.0247679

162. Halcomb E, Fernandez R, Mursa R, Stephen C, Calma K, Ashley C, et al. Mental health, safety and support during COVID-19: A cross-sectional study of primary health care nurses. J Nurs Manag. 2022;30(2):393-402. DOI: 10.1111/jonm.13534

163. Halcomb E, Fernandez R, Mursa R, Stephen C, Calma K, Ashley C, et al. Evaluation of the Brief Coping Orientation to Problems Experienced scale and exploration of coping among primary health care nurses during COVID-19. J Nurs Manag. 2022;30(7):2597-2608. DOI:10.1111/jonm.1381

ANNEX 1

Perceived Stress Scale (PSS-14)

In the last month (or week), how often...	Never	Almost never	Sometimes	Almost always	Always
1. You've been sad about something that happened unexpectedly?					
2. You've felt unable to control important things in your life?					
3. Have you been feeling nervous and "stressed"?					
4. You have dealt successfully of life's difficult problems?*					
5. Do you feel you are coping well with the changes taking place in your life?*					
6. Do you feel confident in your ability to solve personal problems?*					
7. Do you feel that things are happening according to his will?*					
8. You thought you couldn't cope with all the things you have to do?					
9. You've managed to control irritation in your life?*					
10. You feel that things are under your control?*					
11. You've been getting angry because things that happen are out of your control?					
12. Have you found yourself thinking about the things you should do?					
13. Have you been able to control the way you spend your time?					
14. Do you feel that difficulties are accumulate to the point where you believe you can't overcome them?					

* Questions with inverted punctuation

ANNEX 2

Brunel Humour Scale (BRUMS)

How have you been feeling this last month?	Nothing	A little	Moderately	Quite a lot	Extremely
1. Terrified					
2. Lively					
3. Confused					
4. Out of stock					
5. Depressed					
6. Discouraged					
7. Angry					
8. Exhausted					
9. Insecure					
10. Sleepy					
11. Angry					
12. Sad					
13. Anxious					
14. Worried					
15. In the mood					
16. Unhappy					
17. Disorientated					
18. Tension					
19. Angry					
20. With energy					
21. Tired					
22. Grumpy					
23. Alert					
24. Undecided					

Brief Cope

How have you reacted to the stressful situations you've been through?	I haven't done it at all	I've been doing a bit	I've been doing more or less	I've been doing a lot
1) I've been working or doing other things activities to distract me.				
2. I have focussed my efforts on doing something about the situation in which I find myself. meeting.				
3. I've been saying to myself: "This isn't real".				
4. Have I used alcohol or other drugs / medicines to make me feel better.				
5. I have received emotional support from others people.				
6. I'm giving up on the situation.				
7. Have I taken any action to try improve the situation.				
8. I have refused to believe that this situation has happened.				
9. I've been saying things to vent my unpleasant feelings.				
10. I have received help and advice from other people.				
11. Have I used alcohol or other drugs to help me get through the situation.				
12. I've been trying to see the situation differently way to make it seem more positive.				
13. I've been criticising myself.				
14. I've been trying to create a strategy in what to do.				
15. I have received comfort and understanding from someone.				
16. I'm giving up trying to face situation.				
17. I've been trying to see some good in what is happening.				
18. I've been making jokes about the situation.				

19. I've been doing things to think less about the situation, like going to the cinema, watching TV, dreaming awake, sleep or go shopping.				
20. I have accepted the reality of what has happened				
21. I've been expressing my negative feelings.				
22. I've been trying to find comfort in my religion or spiritual beliefs				
23. I've been trying to get advice or help from other people about what to do.				
24. I've learnt to live with the situation.				
25. I've been thinking a lot about the steps I'm going to give.				
26. I've been blaming myself for the things happened.				
27. I've been praying or meditating.				
28. I've been ridiculing the situation				

ANNEX 4

Spiritual Well-being Scale (SWS)

For each of the statements below, choose the best option that indicates how much you agree or disagree with the statement as a description of your personal experience	I agree totally (CT)	I agree partially (CP)	I agree more than disagree (CD)	I disagree more than agree (DC)	I disagree partially (SD)	I disagree totally (DT)
1. I don't find much satisfaction in prayer personal with God*						
2. I don't know who I am, where I came from or where I'm going where I'm going*						
3. I believe that God loves and cares for me with me						
4. I feel that life is a positive experience						
5. I believe that God is impersonal and is not is interested in my everyday situations*						
6. I feel uneasy about my future*						
7. I have a meaningful personal relationship with God						
8. I feel very fulfilled and satisfied with life						
9. I don't get much personal strength and support from my God*						
10. I have a sense of well-being about the direction my life is taking						
11. I believe that God cares about my problems						
12. I don't enjoy life very much*						
13. I don't have a satisfactory personal relationship with God*						
14. I feel good about my future						
15. My relationship with God helps me not feel alone						
16. I feel that life is full of conflicts and unhappiness*						
17. I feel fully realised when I am in intimate communion with God						
18. Life doesn't have much meaning*						
19. My relationship with God contributes to my sense of well-being						
20. I believe there is some real purpose for my life						

* Questions with inverted punctuation

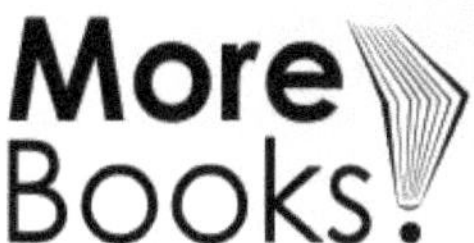
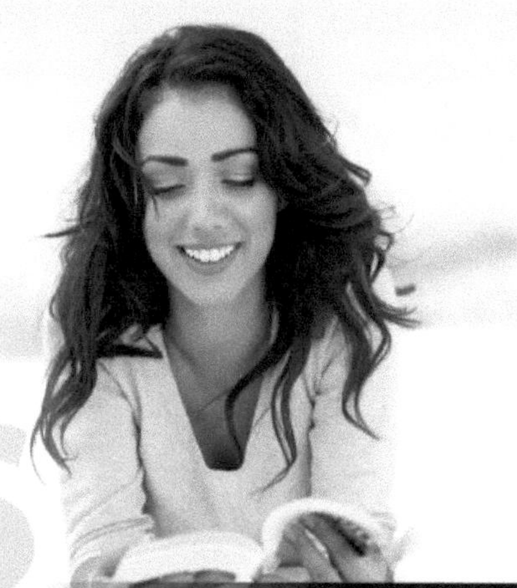

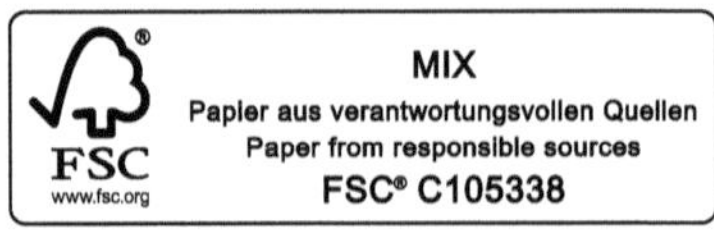

Printed by Books on Demand GmbH, Norderstedt / Germany